Praise from Me~~ltdown Participants~~

"The lifestyle changes I made a[...] [...] [...]appier, and healthier, not to mention th[...]
—*Sirci Kitir, J. C. Penne[...]*

"Carole demonstrated how an average person—who lost weight, got fit, and went public—can indeed change hundreds of lives."
—*Lew Sitzer, Executive Director, Nevada County Television*

"The Meltdown was just what I needed—it was so inspiring."
—*Sue Munson, Receptionist, Family Practice Office*

"I have struggled with being overweight my whole life. Today I know there is no magic pill . . . Although I haven't yet reached my goal, I've made healthy changes."
—*Kerry Arnett, Former Mayor, Nevada City*

"Each person on our team worked at whatever program was best for them. Everyone was feeding off everyone else's success."
—*Susanna Trevena, Bank Executive, Citizens Bank of Northern California*

"My whole body is healthier—not just my knees and heart but also my spirit. Being around people struggling with the same fitness issues was encouraging! Tackling the issues together sparked my enthusiasm."
—*Patti Wood, Teacher's Assistant*

"Our country has many cities, but few communities. Today, we have a great sense of community."
—*Susan Kopp, Clerk of the Court of Nevada County*

"Dieting isn't new to me . . . Then along comes this crazy community event, the Meltdown. I never had a support system of a thousand people before."
—*Ann Mitchell, Elementary School Teacher*

"One thing the Meltdown did was plant the idea that there's no reason to wait to do things you want to do."
—*Molly Fisk, Poet*

"From the restaurants that offered special menus to grocery stores offering Meltdown recipes, business owners found their own unique way to participate and contribute to the cause of fitness."
—*Mary Ann Mueller, President/CEO, Grass Valley/Nevada County Chamber*

"We did not register to be part of the official Meltdown . . .Together, our [secret] team—husband, 65; wife, 62; and married daughter, 35—lost over sixty pounds."
—*"Dick, Mary, and Jane Doe"—Too Private to Go Public*

"One of my biggest pleasures was seeing my eighty-two-year-young mom enjoy the [Meltdown] so much. She just missed being the biggest winner for weight loss."
—*Mary Baron, Realtor*

"I now have four friends I would have never met . . . if it hadn't been for the Meltdown!"
—*Beverly Cooper, Retired Marketing Director*

"My new scale and I are becoming good friends. All that I learned through the Meltdown continues to help me on my journey to becoming a healthier me."
—*Dena Nick, Homemaker*

"The Meltdown gave me a sense of strength and balance not only for my workouts, but also in life."
—*Alisha Randall, High School Student*

"All my life I have fought my weight. At last I was part of a team in an extremely large group of people with the same frustrations, questions, and concerns. The meetings were fun and exciting! And the excitement was contagious!"
—*Carol Marquis, Homemaker*

Doctors and Others Recommend the Meltdown as an Rx for Fitness

"I know all too well the pain associated with being seriously overweight. Unfortunately, it's something that way too many people struggle with. The solution is that each of us must take the first step on the sacred journey to fitness and find the pathway to health and wellness that matches our unique lifestyle. *From Fat to Fit* will give you the inspiration and courage to begin. And begin we must—while we still can."
> —*Nicholas "Dr. Nick" Yphantides, MD, Author,* My Big Fat Greek Diet

"An inspiring story of a personal transformation that spread to an entire community. It shows that weight loss doesn't have to be a solitary activity and can actually be fun when others are involved. *From Fat to Fit* offers a blueprint for other towns to follow."
> —*Edward Abramson, PhD, Author,* Body Intelligence

"Carole shows the power of one person to transform a community. Her personal story inspired thousands of others to take action and get healthy, and this book shows how you too can be a catalyst for change in yourself and your community."
> —*Nedra Kline Weinreich, President, Weinreich Communications*

"Carole Carson not only walks her talk and puts her smart calorie count where her mouth is, she is the Pied Piper of fitness, leading an entire town on the road to health."
> —*Mel Walsh, Author,* Hot Granny

"This program proves that fun and friendship, values so integral to the Red Hat Society (a women's social organization) can also provide invaluable support in the pursuit of physical fitness."
> —*Sue Ellen Cooper, Founder, Red Hat Society*

"If you are ready to take responsibility for your own health, Carole and Meltdown participants offer inspiration."
> —*Christine Newsom, MD, Internal Medicine*

"Carole Carson brilliantly shows us that with intention, structure, and committed action, anything is possible; she invites us to declare our dreams and bring them into reality. This book is a must-read for anyone interested in creating lasting health."

—*Maxine Barish-Wreden, MD, and Kay Judge, MD, Co-Medical Directors, Sutter Heart Institute, Women's Heart Advantage*

"After reading this book, there is no way that one will be able to ignore what we put in our bodies, the fact that some type of regular exercise must be integrated into our daily routine, and the knowledge our future quality of life will be defined by the decisions we make today."

—*Lloyd Dean, President and CEO, Catholic Healthcare West*

"*From Fat to Fit* is a must-read for anyone who works with families and children. Parents can experience the joy of helping their whole family live longer, healthier, and happier lives. This fun-filled and easy-to-read book shows us how."

—*Mardie Caldwell, COAP, Founder, Lifetime Adoption; Talk Show Host; Author, Award-winning Book* AdoptingOnline.com

"We are increasingly aware of the impact of lifestyle choices on long-term well-being. Through better eating and regular exercise, individuals can improve their cardiovascular health. This book encourages readers to take their first steps in this direction."

—*John A. Mallery, MD, Cardiologist*

"Thank you for sharing this wonderful achievement in *From Fat to Fit*. This fabulous piece of work will inspire many of the citizens of our state."

—*Durand "Rudy" Macklin, Director, Bureau of Minority Health, State of Louisiana*

"One of those rare moments when ordinary people working together do something extraordinary. It made a lasting impression."

—*Jeff Ackerman, Publisher,* The Union

FROM FAT TO FIT

Turn Yourself into a Weapon of MASS REDUCTION

Carole Carson

WARNING

Reading this book may dramatically improve your lifestyle.
Possible side effects: A sudden impulse to get fit and make friends!

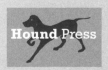

Hound Press

The articles and profiles of individuals appearing in this book were originally published in their entirety in the *Union* newspaper (www.theunion.com). Unattributed quotations are written by Carole Carson. Use of photographs on pages 7, 10, 14, 18, 22, 26, 30, 40, 44, 48, 52, 56, 61, 66, 70, 74, 77, 82, 95, 100, 106, 112, 116, 118, 133 (bottom), and 140 is provided courtesy of the *Union* newspaper. The photographs on pages 1, 89, 119, 125, 153, 173, 177, 184, 187, 192, and 195 are reprinted with permission of Larry Scott. The photographs on pages 134 and 186 are reprinted with permission of Friendship Club. The photograph on page 147 is reprinted with permission of Kathy Palmer. The photograph on page 122 is reprinted with permission of Mike Carville. The photograph on page 35 is reprinted with permission of Steve Lurie. The photographs on pages 132 (left), 135, 148, 156, 159, 160, 164, 166, 167, 169, and 189 are reprinted with permission of Marc Lurie.

Hound Press
P.O. Box 2328, Nevada City, CA 95959
Tel: (530) 478-5709   Fax: (530) 478-1108   www.HoundPress.com

Ordering Information

Quantity sales. Special discounts are available on quantity purchases by corporations, associations, and others. For details, contact the "Special Sales Department" at the Hound Press address above.

Individual sales. Hound Press publications are available through most bookstores. They can also be ordered directly from Hound Press: Tel: (866) 337-7836; Fax: (530) 478-1108; www.HoundPress.com.

Orders by U.S. trade bookstores and wholesalers. Please contact Independent Publishers Group, 814 North Franklin Street, Chicago, IL 60610 Tel: (312) 337-0747; Fax (312) 337-5983.

Printed in the United States of America

Interior design by Sue Knopf, Graffolio

Cataloging-in-Publication Data

Carson, Carole Louise.
   From fat to fit : turn yourself into a weapon of mass reduction / Carole Carson.
   p. cm.
   1ˢᵗ edition.
   Includes bibliographical references and index.
   ISBN 10: 0-9766030-9-8; ISBN-13: 978-0-9766030-9-2
   1. Weight loss 2. Health. 3. Physical fitness. I. Title.
RM222.2 .C326 2007
613.2519--dc22   2006936328

First Edition
12 11 10 09 08 07   10 9 8 7 6 5 4 3 2 1

DISCLAIMER

This book provides information on how to make lifestyle changes for greater fitness. It is sold with the understanding that neither the publisher nor author is rendering medical, psychiatric, or other professional services. For expert assistance, the services of a competent professional should be sought.

This book encourages individuals and communities to become more fit. The author and Hound Press shall assume neither liability nor responsibility to any person or entity with respect to any damage caused, or alleged to have been caused, directly, or indirectly, by information provided in this book. If you do not wish to be bound by the above, you may return the book within thirty (30) days of purchase, together with proof of purchase, to the publisher for a full refund.

Contents

Foreword: What's at Stake? vii

Part 1: The Accidental Journalist 1

Week 1: Just Undo It! 9

Week 2: Starting to Change 13

Week 3: Eating to Live, Not Living to Eat 17

Week 4: Giving Birth to the New Me 21

Week 5: Counting the Cost 25

Week 6: Running the Gauntlet—Feasting in France 29

Week 7: Why Don't French Women Get Fat? 33

Week 8: The Lull before the Storm 39

Week 9: Everything Changes 43

Week 10: You Gotta Have Friends 47

Week 11: What Does It Take? 51

Week 12: The More I Lose, the More of "Me" There Is 55

Week 13: Entering the Home Stretch 59

Week 14: On the Road Again 65

Week 15: Nothing Tastes as Good as Being Thinner Feels 69

Week 16: From Shame to Joy 73

Part 2: Learning as I Go—Continuing the Journey 77

Am I Crazy Enough to Think I Can Change the World? 81

Suffering First-Degree Burns While Carrying the Torch of Fitness . . 85

Wrestling with Devils 91

Relearning the Three Rs 97

A Matter of Life and Death 103

Pride Goeth before a Fall 109

When the Apple Is Ripe 113

Part 3: From a Private to a Public Matter 119

The Nevada County Meltdown Takes Shape 123

Week 1: Riding the Tiger 131

Week 2: Achieving Our Personal Best 137

Week 3: The Circle Keeps Expanding 145

Week 4: Beaming Our Message Beyond 155

Week 5: From Fat City to Tiny Town 163

Week 6: The Tail Wags the Dog 171

Week 7: A Lid for Every Pot 175

Week 8: The Best Is Yet to Come! 181

Getting off the Tiger and onto a Bigger One 191

Part 4: Proliferating Weapons of Mass Reduction 195

Up Close and Personal: Getting Fit Together 199

Take the Leap: Seven Steps to Personal Fitness 205

Run with the Big Dogs! Seven Steps to Community Fitness . . 211

What Have You Got to Lose? What Have You Got to Gain? . . 217

Appendices 219

Appendix A: Fifty-six Discoveries about Eating and Cooking . . . 221

Appendix B: Web Site Resources 229

Index 239

Acknowledgments 243

About the Author 247

*The greatest discovery of my generation
is that a human being can alter his life
by altering his attitudes of mind.*

WILLIAM JAMES

What's at Stake?

By now almost all of us can recite the statistics: Nearly two-thirds of adult Americans are overweight. Half of these overweight Americans are obese—thirty or more pounds overweight. Lack of fitness now challenges tobacco as the leading cause of preventable death. Obese adults have a 50 to 100 percent increased risk of premature death. Evidently, robust old age and obesity are not on speaking terms.

Children learn from adults. A national health and nutrition survey reveals that 15 percent of young people are overweight and thus at risk of diabetes and high cholesterol. With an obese parent, these children also have an 80 percent chance of becoming obese adults.

Such children face a triple whammy:

- Reduced odds of ever enjoying normal weight

- Painful social discrimination from being overweight

- Significantly increased risk of medical problems potentially resulting in a shorter life span than that of their parents

Besides causing personal distress, obesity-induced medical problems challenge the medical care delivery system and are certain to become a financial drain on future generations.

Mary Simmonds, MD, president of the American Cancer Society, says, "Up to one-third of cancer deaths are related to diet and the lack of physical activity." Moreover, the list of medical problems associated with obesity continues to grow—from heart disease, stroke, and diabetes to Alzheimer's disease and infertility.

The National Center for Chronic Disease Prevention and Health Promotion estimates 300,000 premature deaths from obesity each year. About $177 billion is spent on directly related medical costs. Indirect costs such as absenteeism, disability, reduced productivity, and increased medical premiums are absorbed by employers. A recent study in California suggests that the annual cost to the state's economy for inactive, overweight, and obese adults is $28 billion. Extending this cost to fifty states reveals the magnitude of the public health problem.

Although these numbers should press us into action, they are difficult to grasp. Abstract and boring, the calculations of experts seem unrelated to our day-to-day lives. We need to remind ourselves that behind the statistics are the personal stories of much needless suffering, distress, or death—not of strangers but of family members, friends, even ourselves.

The epidemic of obesity is now global. The World Health Organization reports that over a billion adults are overweight, far more than the 600 million who are undernourished. And the problem grows. In 1995, the World Health Organization classified 200 million adults as obese. Today, the number is 300 million. Referring to "globesity," WHO considers it an obvious yet painfully neglected worldwide public health issue. Ironically, right along with efforts to eliminate malnutrition and starvation, WHO is also trying to organize a global response to obesity.

Whether because of lifestyle changes (spending more time sitting in our cars commuting, watching television, or working at a desk) or because of accessible food everywhere (at the touch of a finger on the microwave or by voice command at a drive-through microphone), we are getting dangerously fat.

Lack of fitness is visible everywhere—in schools, workplaces, doctors' offices, hospitals, and ultimately in supersized caskets. We've got it backwards—instead of doing more and eating less, we are eating more and doing less!

Looking into the future, we do not see a quick cure on the horizon. Unlike smallpox—virtually eliminated through vaccination—obesity and lack of fitness have no simple remedy. There is no vaccination for the consequences of our choices.

Even more troublesome is our approach to the problem as a purely private and often embarrassing issue. Many of us, especially women, find it easier to talk about our sex life to a stranger than reveal our weight to our spouse!

Such a mindset carries a double burden. Not only are we fat, but to have gotten this way we must also be weak willed. Except for rare chats with one's physician or perhaps a close friend, fat issues remain locked up in a private box of secret recriminations. Popular culture—in magazines, on television, at workplaces, in schools—reminds us daily that "thin is beautiful" and "fat is unattractive." It is a message that compounds personal shame.

Surprisingly, private needs and public interests occasionally intersect. That's what happened in our community! One woman, Carole Carson, came out of the closet, courageously breaking the taboo of silence. On the front page of the local newspaper, she openly admitted her shame and guilt about being obese and out of shape. She made a public commitment to share the experience of going from fat to fit.

I have been a nurse for twenty-five years, and my job and passion require counseling people about healthy lifestyles, including weight loss. Because Carole's makeover represented an opportunity to motivate others, I contacted her and offered my services—an initial health risk assessment and ongoing clinical guidance. Over the course of sixteen weeks, I witnessed her transformation from fat to fit.

As I had hoped, when readers saw an ordinary person making changes, they realized they could experience similar success.

Later, when Carole invited others to join her in getting fit through a community program—the Nevada County Meltdown—neighbors and friends responded by the hundreds. Our community, sharing in the personal shame of not being fit, discovered that we urgently needed to make healthier choices.

Our private needs and our public interests were one.

Creating new bonds, we built a community around a common goal— living healthier. Strangers shared intimacy and candor. Status, religion, and political affiliation became irrelevant. A manicurist teamed up with a truck driver, a stay-at-home mom, a nurse, and a retiree. The glue? A commitment to fitness!

The results were spectacular.

Individuals who had previously struggled with weight loss and fitness suddenly were joined by friends and neighbors—all with the same challenges—seeking to accomplish together what they could not do by themselves.

They discovered that getting fit was fun! And together they set out to change their lives. Together they cheered their triumphs. Together they discovered that the old seesaw patterns of dieting were over. Because they were doing it together, they found a completely new path to weight loss—a way of life combining friendship and fitness.

Local businesses were quick to capitalize on this community-based issue. Health and fitness clubs offered free use of facilities to registered participants. Restaurants introduced Meltdown entrees on updated menus. Grocery stores promoted fruits and vegetables and low-calorie cookbooks. Kitchenware stores provided discounts on appliances and tools to achieve lower-calorie cooking. Local businesses were finding ways to satisfy their customers' desires for a healthier lifestyle.

Working together, more than a thousand people lost nearly four tons in seven weeks. They shared no common diet or plan. Devotees of Weight Watchers, no-carb dieters, vegetarians, raw foodists, and others combined ideas for changing the ways they ate.

Participants worked out in gyms, walked baby llamas, or did yoga. Some jogged while others hiked or bicycled or played tennis. Some attended aerobic or Jazzercise classes while others walked in a pool, gardened, or worked out to a videotape.

No single exercise or diet was recommended or promoted. Instead, participants were encouraged to achieve fitness in their own unique ways—whatever worked for them and could be permanently integrated into their lives.

Despite these differing approaches, the group shared a solid commitment to fitness, a thread of commitment that wove together hundreds. These same people worked closely for eight weeks to share the significant changes they were experiencing. Dozens more, though not registered, participated vicariously through spouses, friends, family members, or fellow employees.

Depicting the struggles, insights, and momentum, Carole's book tells the story, from her own personal transformation—from fat to fit—to the dilemmas and struggles of others who wanted, needed, sometimes desperately, to lead a healthier life.

To the surprise of everyone, including Carole, a whole community came together in the Meltdown, as it came to be known. As people jumped in to lend energy and time, the event increasingly took on a life of its own.

Carole, viewing herself as an ordinary person who lost weight, got fit, and went public, significantly helped to dramatically change a community.

Whether you want to become more fit or want to help others lead healthier lives, you will discover it is easier than you think, for yourself and for your community. You've taken the first step by picking up this book.

Debbie Wagner, RN
Director of Occupational Health and Wellness
Sierra Nevada Memorial Hospital
Nevada County, California

PART 1

The Accidental Journalist

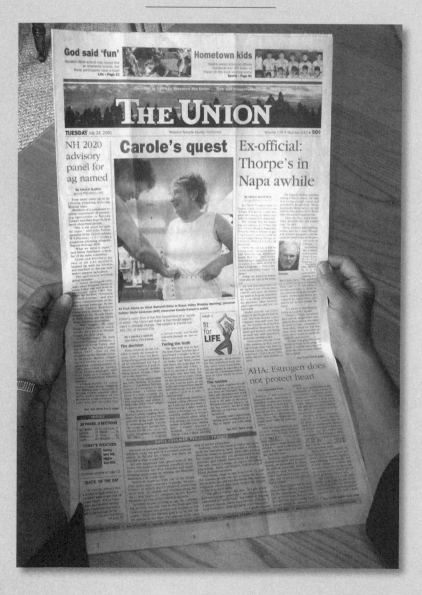

Courage is being scared to death—
but saddling up anyway.

JOHN WAYNE

) (

I stepped out of the shower. Unwilling to put on underwear because it might add an extra ounce or two, I stood naked on the bathroom scale. Sucking in my stomach and holding my breath, I waited for the number that would determine my outlook for the day.

Yesterday, my 5'1" frame registered 179 pounds. Size 16 clothes were tight. A few size 18 tops had sneaked into my closet.

What would today bring? No number appeared on the scale. I stepped on and off the scale several times before realizing the scale was broken. Was there a message here?

Disheartened, I looked up, half expecting God's voice to break through the ceiling. The bathroom was quiet; I heard only my own voice, filled with self-loathing.

"How could you have gotten this fat?"

The next morning I went through the same ritual with a new and more accurate scale. Now I weighed 182—three pounds more!

"That's it!" I said, more in desperation than conviction. "If you don't change, you'll die fat. You have to do something before it's too late!"

Even though I didn't know where to begin and had failed hundreds of times in the past, I allowed myself the tiniest ray of hope. As tough as making changes would be, nothing could be worse than the verbal beatings I was giving myself.

Every day the voice incessantly nagged at me: "How could you let yourself get this fat?" "Why are you so weak-willed?" If self-loathing and shame were measurable, I had soared to the ninety-ninth percentile.

Shopping for clothes was a nightmare. I'd leave the changing room so determined to lose weight that I'd skip lunch, only to rebound and overeat that night.

Repeated failures had taught me one important lesson—wanting to change and actually changing are two different things. No question that I wanted to change, but would I? Could I?

Looking back, I realized my problem: I had tried to do it alone. For the first time, I admitted that I needed help.

Over breakfast I noticed a newspaper article suggesting fitness coaches weren't just for rich people. Maybe I could start there, I thought.

I began calling gyms to interview trainers. Since I was sporting a hamstring badly torn from trying to play tennis while out of shape, my near-term ability to exercise was limited. Maybe a little walking in the lap pool or some upper-body exercises? Since I'd never worked out in a gym with weights and resistance machines, I had no idea where to begin. For sure, though, I didn't want to reinjure my leg.

After several phone interviews, one trainer's style particularly appealed to me. Gayle Lossman laughed even more than I did. Her voice also sounded seasoned and mature. In talking with her, I realized I didn't want to work with an anorexic bimbette who had yet to bear the stretch marks of motherhood. When I told her how much I weighed and how out of shape I was, Gayle wasn't judgmental. Just the opposite—she seemed genuinely enthusiastic about my makeover project.

Later, when we met at a local gym, I discovered she was my age. One look at her stunning figure, and I blurted out, "Whatever you're doing, I want to do that too!"

Gayle insisted we set a specific goal for a certain amount of time. Since my sixtieth birthday was four months away, I said I wanted to lose forty pounds in four months. I had no idea if that was reasonable or not, but the numbers sounded symmetrical.

Two weeks into my new lifestyle and reasonably confident I'd follow through, I contacted the local newspaper and asked the assignment editor if an article on a senior citizen getting fit might be useful.

I'd already written a couple of travel articles for our small-town newspaper, the *Union*, which covered events in our section of the Sierra foothills. With fewer than 20,000 residents in our two adjacent towns, Grass Valley and Nevada City, and 80,000 people scattered throughout the rest of the county, the *Union* was the main source of local news.

Somehow the paper managed to bridge the various elements in our community, reaching descendents of the Cornish miners who came looking for gold, aging San Francisco hippies who later became artists and business owners, and newly retired professionals from Los Angeles and the Bay Area, like me. Given the rural nature of the county, the newspaper also reported on topics of interest to ranchers and farmers. Even criminals had their section where their daily activities—mostly petty crimes and vandalism—were reported in detail.

Thinking there might be other seniors who needed to shape up, I e-mailed the editor with an offer to write a one-time piece on the theme of "you're never too old to get fit." If accepted, the article would appear in the Wednesday senior section. The back of the newspaper suited me just fine.

To my delight, the editor wanted the piece and arranged for an accompanying photograph to be taken at the gym where I worked out.

With the photographer snapping away, Gayle took my measurements. Although the photograph revealed my girth, she and I conspired to make sure the numbers on the scale were hidden. We also tried unsuccessfully to hide the numbers on the measuring tape around my waist—forty-four inches.

On Monday night I received an unexpected phone call from the assignment editor.

"Would you mind," she asked, "if we ran the article Tuesday instead of Wednesday? Tuesdays are usually slow news days."

Then, as if an afterthought, she added, "Oh, and by the way, we might want to make this a series, maybe show some photographs and get some comments from you along the way."

I couldn't think of any reason to object, so I agreed. The request struck me as odd, though, because the senior section only ran on Wednesdays. *Where else might they place the article?* I wondered. As for a future article, I'd wait and see.

Crawling into bed that night, I couldn't help asking, *What was the connection between Tuesday being a slow news day and my article?* Then the terrible thought occurred, *What if the article appeared on the front page with my weight and measurements for everyone in town to see?* An involuntary shudder passed through my body. I was sick to my stomach. Suddenly I was struck by the worst anxiety attack of my life.

I tried reassuring myself that a fat person going on a diet was hardly front-page news, even for a small-town newspaper. The logic was unassailable, but the anxiety wouldn't go away. I slept fitfully.

At 5:00 AM, the sound of a phone rudely awakened me. It was Gayle. "Have you seen the morning paper?" she asked laughingly.

I felt the pit in the bottom of my stomach grow.

"Go get it," she barked. "We're on the front page."

With dread mounting by the second, I didn't take time to get dressed. Instead I threw on my bathrobe and drove the half mile to our mailbox.

Not until I was safely home and inside the house did I carefully unfold the newspaper. My worst fears materialized! A huge color picture, front and center, revealed my obesity for the whole world to see. At 182 pounds, I looked like a large, yellow, overstuffed canary with a forty-four-inch waist.

I tried to grasp the implications. Everyone—my neighbors, my friends downtown, everyone!—would know my measurements and weight. Oh, my God—even my husband! I'd always hidden my weight from him. Not that he cared—he loved me however I looked. For years, though, I hadn't been honest with the Department of Motor Vehicles. If someone in their office saw the newspaper, would I lose my driver's license?

There was only one solution.

Impatiently I waited for my husband to come downstairs and join me for breakfast. Pushing the paper across the table, I hit him with the decision.

"We have to move," I said. And I meant it.

Later in the day, errands took me to town. I dreaded seeing anyone—especially anyone I knew—certain that contact would result in further humiliation.

To my surprise, the opposite occurred. "Go for it, Carole," I heard from the grocery clerk who checked my groceries and the receptionist at my doctor's office.

Everywhere I went, people came forward and shared their misery, confessing how they were struggling with the same problem. When I protested that I wouldn't have written the article if I had known it would appear on the front page, they still commended my courage.

When I stopped by to visit friends during their regularly scheduled tennis clinic, our coach teased me about the publicity.

"Carole goes on a diet, and it's front-page news," he said laughingly.

My feelings weren't hurt. I knew that despite the teasing, he was pleased at my overdue commitment to shape up. Both of us knew that I wouldn't have fallen and torn my hamstring if I hadn't been carrying around so much extra weight.

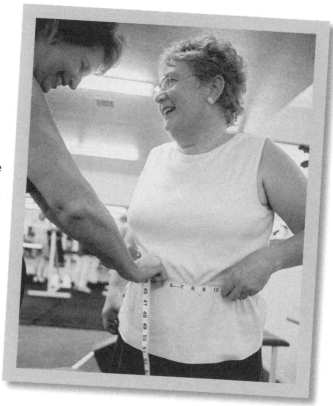

Here I am for the whole world to see—the fattest I've ever been in my life!

Even so, I had to admit it did seem odd to have the article appear on the front page right next to important news stories. Was there a larger purpose to be served?

With all the comments from strangers and good-humored ribbing from tennis friends, I came home in a state of exhilaration. By publicly admitting my lack of fitness, I'd accidentally broken a taboo that evidently haunted others as much as me. Coming out of the closet as I did gave them the freedom to tell me about their shame and embarrassment. Equally important, I had inadvertently solicited support—something I'd never even thought of asking for before.

Having gone this far, I would stay the course. Each week, for the next sixteen weeks, I would expose my ups and downs, my progress and lapses, my measurements and weight, and even my thoughts as I reinvented myself. I'd experiment with different forms of exercise and address a new eating style to help me reach my ideal weight.

Chronicling my own experience might be useful to others. Plus, it would give me perspective on this life-altering experience. One thing for sure: it would keep me honest.

Almost magically, fear and loathing disappeared, replaced by a sense of adventure.

That night, still mulling over what I'd said at breakfast, my husband asked me where I wanted to move.

"Move?" I indignantly responded. "We can't move. I have a newspaper series to write!"

Just Undo It!

A bad habit never disappears miraculously;
it's an undo-it-yourself project.
ABIGAIL VAN BUREN

I needed to begin the newspaper series with an honest accounting of how I had come to this turning point. Stepping back a little, I realized that three events in my life collided to push me toward fitness. First, I had just been injured. Besides healing my torn hamstring, I wanted to stay injury free so I could pursue a lifelong dream of playing competitive tennis.

Second, I was approaching my sixtieth birthday. Even though I was energetic and active, I did not like what I saw in the mirror. Being classified as obese was depressing enough without the prospect of gaining even more weight in the coming year.

Third was my doctor's subtle nagging about my high cholesterol, high blood pressure, and slowly increasing weight. The combination of tennis, vanity, and health concerns made me sure that this time I needed to take action.

Facing the Truth

What pushed me over the top, though, was facing the truth. Naked in my own bathroom, I saw the number on the scale reach 182 pounds.

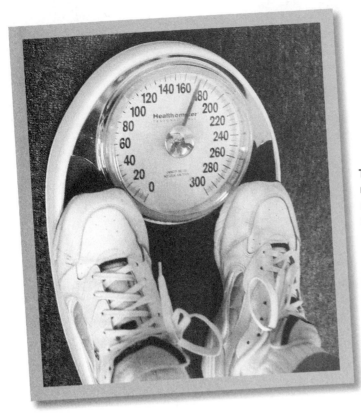

The scale numbers are starting to go down—a first in a long time!

Even worse was my girth. Those numbers that Gayle and I measured had bulked up over the years in fractions of inches at a time. It was the same way I would need to take them off.

The Program Schedule

The exercise plan Gayle set up for me took into account both my goals and my limitations. To build upper-body strength, on Mondays, Wednesdays, and Fridays I would work with Gayle in the weight room in a local gym for one hour. On Tuesdays, Thursdays, and Saturdays I would walk in an indoor pool for thirty minutes, or less if my hamstring complained. With healing, the level and amount of exercise would be increased and lower-body routines would be added.

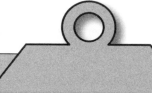

Progress Report
Week 1

Description	Start 7/13	Now 7/20	Goal 11/2	Result to Date
Weekly exercise	2 hrs/wk	7 hrs/wk	12 hrs/wk	Increased 5 hrs/wk
Weight	179	174	139	Lost 5 pounds
Total measurements*	381	374	341	Lost 7 inches

*Total measurements include neck, chest, bust, upper torso, waist, hips, upper thighs, lower thighs, upper arms, lower arms, calves, wrists, ankles.

Progress When I made my unequivocal decision to get fit, I weighed 182 pounds. I had ten days before I began my weekly reports. I used the time to lose 3 pounds. During my first "official" week beginning July 13, I lost 5 more pounds. Already my clothes fit better.

My weekly chronicle ends November 2, three days before my sixtieth birthday. What a nice present for myself!

Obstacles Surprise! Jury duty summons! Can I fit everything in?

Goals

When Gayle pushed me to set goals, I could think only of my upcoming sixtieth birthday. I could set a modest goal for then and feel confident about reaching it. Or I could go for my dream. I chose the latter, knowing it would be a stretch.

By my sixtieth birthday I wanted a completely rehabilitated leg. Even more, I wanted new habits that could sustain a lifetime of fitness.

As a by-product of the first two goals, I also wanted healthy cholesterol and blood pressure and to be well on my way toward losing forty pounds.

Fear of Failure Sets In

Of course, as soon as I set my goals, fear of failure set in. Could I actually change after all these years? Fitness isn't only for the young, I said to reassure myself. A person is never too old to get fit. At fifty-nine, I had more time, resources, and self-discipline than when I was younger. Maturity was a plus. Still I wondered: Was this just brave talk? Would I follow through? Would I revert to my old ways? Time would tell.

Starting to Change

Never eat more than you can lift.
MISS PIGGY

My trainer, Gayle, set fitness guidelines: If I ate 2,500 calories a day (current weight times 15, approximately), I'd maintain my weight. If I ate less and exercised more, I'd lose. A shortfall of 3,500 calories on average equaled one pound. A safe, if ambitious, goal for weight loss was two pounds a week. More than four, and I risked my health.

"Enlightened" Eating

Gayle also made some specific suggestions for eating. Her recommendations were not exactly carefully guarded secrets. In fact, I pretty much already knew what to do. Still, with my sixtieth birthday approaching, it was now or never. And so when Gayle set guidelines for "enlightened" eating, I listened closely:

Timing: Eat three evenly balanced meals a day with three snacks (morning, afternoon, evening). No skipped meals or heavy dinner.

Portions: Keep portions modest. No seconds. Include four ounces of lean protein at each meal to manage appetite. Eat until satisfied—not full. Proportions for typical dinner plate: one-quarter lean protein; one-quarter complex carbohydrate; and one-half vegetables. Dessert is fruit.

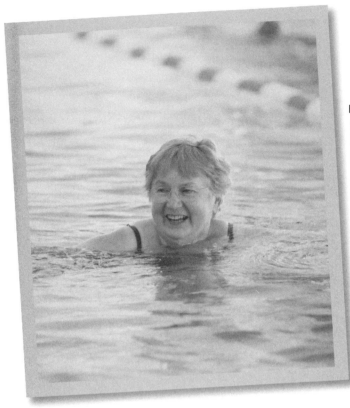

Due to increased resistance, one hour walking in a pool is equivalent to two hours walking on land. Although my walking, even in a pool, is limited by pain in my hamstring, I can laugh as much as I want.

Food Preparation: Broil meat, steam vegetables. (If oil is needed, use olive oil sparingly.)

Choices: Pick a wide variety of foods. Focus on foods high in water (cucumbers or grapes, for example), fiber, minerals, and vitamins and low in fat, sugar, and starch. Take vitamin and calcium supplements. Use whole or unprocessed grains. Without splurging, give yourself one day a week to make one free choice!

Fluids: Drink two glasses of water with every meal. Keep hydrated during exercise periods.

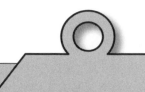

Progress Report
Week 2

Description	Start 7/13	Now 7/27	Goal 11/2	Result to Date
Weekly exercise	2 hrs/wk	8 hrs/wk	12 hrs/wk	Increased 6 hrs/wk
Weight	179	170	139	Lost 9 pounds
Total measurements*	381	365	341	Lost 16 inches

* Total measurements include neck, chest, bust, upper torso, waist, hips, upper thighs, lower thighs, upper arms, lower arms, calves, wrists, ankles.

Progress This week I carefully hit my first tennis balls since tearing my hamstring and increased my exercise time. My eating habits are changing. During the week, I lost nine inches overall and four pounds. I'm thrilled. Wherever I go, there are lots of conversations with people in the same boat.

Obstacles I must remember to focus on fitness, not just losing weight. I must focus on this week, this day. "One healthy choice at a time. One healthy choice at a time." This will be my mantra.

Difficult Beginning

I started putting Gayle's guidelines into action. I began to pay attention, while eating, to when I felt satisfied but not full. I tried to stop eating at that point. To make sure I wasn't overeating, I slowed down, even to the point of putting my fork down between bites. I wanted to give my body time to send a message before I had overeaten.

I also began keeping a food diary, writing down what I had eaten to keep track of calories. The allowance was 1,200 calories a day. Because of a tendency to underestimate the amount of calories in food—partly as the result of denial and partly because of portion size—I set my goal for 1,100. It was a cautious but necessary strategy since most days I typically reached 1,200 calories, even with careful monitoring.

The changes were a shock to my system. Like many overweight people, I loved to cook and eat. Food was my recreational drug of choice. Raised on a farm, I liked meat-centered meals, real butter, and desserts. I also wanted to eat my heaviest meal at night.

The most difficult part was giving up those stuporous evening meals complete with dessert. Already in the first weeks of my new eating style, that afternoon energy bar and nightly bowl of bran cereal were becoming lifesavers.

Yet how responsive the body is when we take care of it! By the end of the second week, I could already see changes when I looked in the mirror. I felt empowered. I had no idea that positive results would come so fast. Maybe this time I could make real—and lasting—changes.

Eating to Live, Not Living to Eat

Are you eating it? Or is it eating you?

LARRY COHEN

To keep following Gayle's eating guidelines, I had to make changes, not just in my eating habits, but in how I thought about food. Instead of viewing food as a major source of gratification, I had to learn to see food as a source of fuel and health. Instead of living to eat, I would eat to live.

What Didn't Work: "Going on a Diet"

I knew from past failures what didn't work: "going on a diet." I'd gone on plenty of them and remembered feeling hungry all the time, especially at night. I couldn't skip meals, either; I'd only get a headache. Limiting my food choices, like eating only cabbage for a week, also wouldn't work. Neither would cooking separate dinners for my husband and me or not being able to dine out.

Above all else, "going on a diet" implied the change was temporary. A "diet" meant "rules," which I knew I'd eventually break. This time I was looking for permanent change. Diet meant deprivation; instead, I wanted to enjoy eating.

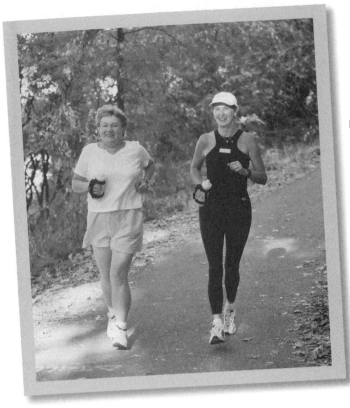

I think Gayle can run forever without being winded. As for me, I can only run a minute before having to walk again.

My Assets

At least I had a few assets: I liked almost all foods. Moreover, I was willing to learn, and I was prepared to give up anything that separated me from fitness.

Plus, this time I was impatient. Whereas before I might have tested the waters one toe at a time, now I was becoming a "just undo it!" person—diving in and getting the shock over with quickly. Impatient for results, I was plunging into significant eating changes.

Feeling the Benefits

Although following Gayle's eating program was tough initially, I soon started to feel as well as see its benefits. I woke up in the morning with

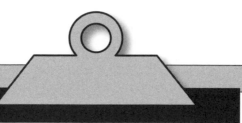

Progress Report
Week 3

Description	Start 7/13	Now 8/3	Goal 11/2	Result to Date
Weekly exercise	2 hrs/wk	9 hrs/wk	12 hrs/wk	Increased 7 hrs/wk
Weight	179	168	139	Lost 11 pounds
Total measurements*	381	359	341	Lost 22 inches

* Total measurements include neck, chest, bust, upper torso, waist, hips, upper thighs, lower thighs, upper arms, lower arms, calves, wrists, ankles.

Progress   I tried walking and jogging this week. I also bench-pressed fifty pounds, which is, I'm told, good for a beginner. I switched to decaf coffee and increased exercise time. This week I lost six inches and two pounds.

Obstacles   I had to back off tennis; the strain was too much for my injured hamstring. My impatience to change forty years of bad habits in a few short weeks gets in the way of enjoying the process. I must remember an old adage: "Go slow to go fast."

more energy. Looking in the mirror gave me an instant charge. The hope I was feeling gave me a renewed sense of youthfulness. I noticed my mind was sharper and I needed less sleep—not to mention the clearer conscience I felt because I was doing the healthy thing. Silencing the constantly critical voice was wonderful; the irritable background static was replaced by a sense of anticipation.

As far as I could tell, the only thing this new eating program required me to give up was a childish, undisciplined freedom to eat anything I wanted, in whatever quantity I wanted, whenever I wanted—a fleeting pleasure at best.

Giving Birth to the New Me

Man's main task in life is to give birth to himself,
to become what he potentially is.

ERICH FROMM

Gayle convinced me to experiment with resistance equipment in the weight room at the gym. She assured me that resistance training would help me regain my college figure. Too many women, she told me, think that lifting weights and using resistance machines are the sole province of men. Or even worse, that if a woman lifts weights, she will bulk up, just as men do.

But that notion was wrong, she reassured me. Lifting weights and working with resistance equipment had a different effect on women's bodies—it sculpted our figures and made us firm and trim.

Although I needed no further encouragement, she told me that in addition to altering the overall symmetry of my body, it would increase my metabolic rate. Fat would be more quickly metabolized, and lean muscle mass would be acquired in ways that even aerobic exercise couldn't match.

Had it not been for this coaching, I would never have worked out in the weight room. I continued to feel a little out of place among the machines and sweaty men, but the benefits were irresistible.

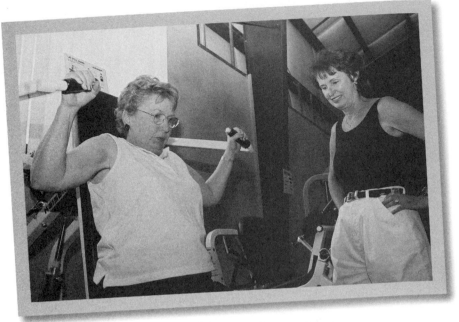

All of this is totally new. If Gayle weren't
coaching me, I'd be too timid to try it.

I still looked like a blimp in the weekly photos, but I was gaining
confidence as well as momentum.

Even so, I awoke in the middle of the night wanting to run away. I
had to remind myself that 2:00 AM was not the best time to make an
important decision. By morning, more of me wanted to continue than
to go back. One day at a time, I told myself.

This week I also did something I had never done before: I signed
up for a 5K walk/run, called the Clydesdale, an event that would be
held a month later at the county fairgrounds. It was Gayle's idea—in
fact, she insisted. I was sure I wouldn't be ready for it. Still, I could feel
a secret excitement growing. What other opportunities had I passed
over because I didn't think I was ready? Maybe getting fit was about
more than just losing weight. Maybe it was about opening up to new
possibilities. Still, I didn't want to embarrass myself in front of everyone.
Would I be ready?

Progress Report
Week 4

Description	Start 7/13	Now 8/10	Goal 11/2	Result to Date
Weekly exercise	2 hrs/wk	10 hrs/wk	12 hrs/wk	Increased 8 hrs/wk
Weight	179	166	139	Lost 13 pounds
Total measurements*	381	356	341	Lost 25 inches

Total measurements include neck, chest, bust, upper torso, waist, hips, upper thighs, lower thighs, upper arms, lower arms, calves, wrists, ankles.

Progress Surprise! I enjoy eating light. Is a thin person struggling to get out? I can't believe I registered for a 5K run/walk—my first ever competitive race. I'm starting to alter or retire clothes. This week I increased my exercise time and lost three inches and two pounds.

Obstacles I lost a dear friend to cancer this week and needed to take time to grieve. Walking is therapy, not just exercise.

Counting the Cost

First say to yourself what you would be;
and then do what you have to do.
EPICTETUS

My decision to get fit had financial implications—I had to pay for a trainer, get some gym clothes, pay membership fees, and potentially replace my wardrobe. To reassure myself that I was worth the money and that we could afford the expense, I talked the matter over with my husband. He suggested that the hidden costs of not being fit were greater. When these costs were calculated, he said, our definition of what was affordable would change.

What's Affordable?

I looked at my recent medical expenses. Over the past two years, high blood pressure and unusual heart sounds had put me in the hospital three times, with thousands of dollars spent on tests and specialists. While our insurance covered much of the cost, we still had paid hundreds of dollars in medical bills. For my torn hamstring—injured because I was out of shape—my insurance company and my husband had coughed up $4,000 for emergency services, hospitalization, doctors, and ambulances.

My husband, who married me in sickness and in health, had started asking, "Where's the health?" With a mounting number of claims, the

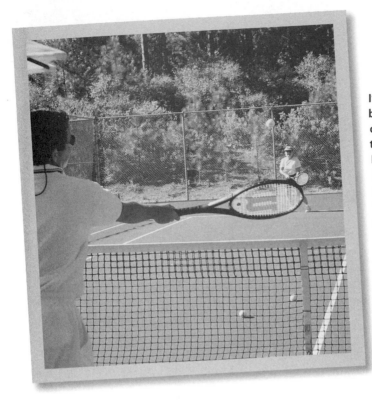

I'm finally back on the court playing tennis. I have a love-hate relationship with the sport: love my good strokes, hate my inconsistency!

medical insurer probably stored my thickening file under C, not for "Carson" but for "Chronic."

Am I Just Getting Old?

Although my illnesses and prescriptions resulted from my choices—I had chosen to be overweight—at the time I considered them a function of aging. For years already I had been noticing aches and pains, especially arthritis in my back and bursitis in my shoulder.

A vague depression had crept into my outlook. I was asking myself, "Am I just getting old?"

Clearly, I had lost the childlike joy of living in my body. Not only that, but long-term I risked being a burden to my family and the health-care system. Possibly I was also shortening my life span.

Progress Report
Week 5

Description	Start 7/13	Now 8/17	Goal 11/2	Result to Date
Weekly exercise	2 hrs/wk	11 hrs/wk	12 hrs/wk	Increased 9 hrs/wk
Weight	179	164	139	Lost 15 pounds
Total measurements*	381	353	341	Lost 28 inches

*Total measurements include neck, chest, bust, upper torso, waist, hips, upper thighs, lower thighs, upper arms, lower arms, calves, wrists, ankles.

Progress Gayle, my trainer, is like a midwife, helping me birth a new, thinner person. She even gives me breathing lessons as I labor in my intense push for fitness. Through our teamwork we have bonded—another unexpected joy. It's ironic, but when I eat less I enjoy my food more. As a special treat, I gingerly hit a few tennis balls, quitting before I reinjured my hamstring. This week I lost three inches and two pounds.

Obstacles Evidently the path to change only has two rules: (1) start and (2) continue. The second rule is the toughest! When I travel to France next week for my son's wedding, can I continue my regimen? I'm a little worried.

The Low-Cost Approach

And so, spurred by articles warning of premature death from lack of fitness, months earlier I had tried the low-cost approach to fitness. I went for a walk alone now and then on a country road near my house. No money needed: the road was free, and I could walk anytime I wanted. The downside was that weather sometimes interfered, walks were limited to daylight hours, and a few times I barely escaped being run over. In addition, I had no support. No one else cared if I skipped my walk. As a result, exercise sessions were sporadic. My low-cost plan produced zilch.

Comparing Costs

This new fitness plan at the outset sounded expensive. Over four months, my husband and I figured out we would spend around $1,600. This included the cost of a trainer for three sessions a week, sixteen weeks of gym-club membership, a pair of running shoes, and miscellaneous gear.

Then we thought about my medical expenses. Over time, we knew we would save at least that much and more on groceries, prescriptions, doctors, and tests. By way of comparison, we had spent at least $1,600 driving and maintaining our car in the previous year; surely my body was as valuable as our automobile!

Priceless

In measuring costs, though, how do we place a value on feeling better and living longer? Or being able to move pain-free with tons of energy? Or looking and feeling younger? Or being able to play tennis? Or reducing the risk of heart disease and cancer?

The rewards were priceless, so the question was not hard to answer. I needed to invest in my body for both current and future dividends. I could only hope it would be the best money I'd ever spend.

Running the Gauntlet— Feasting in France

We are confronted with insurmountable opportunities.

POGO (WALT KELLY)

We flew to Paris and then to Provence for my son's wedding to his delightful French wife. From conversations with him, I knew that her family was making elaborate preparations. Our two weeks would be spent feasting—and, I imagined, in a constant state of self-torture. Among all those beautifully presented foods, wonderful wines, and fabulous desserts, how would I keep my commitment to fitness? Did I even want to? Was this a golden opportunity to escape from my American regimen?

My son's French relatives were surprised to see the "smaller" me. I was already down twenty pounds since we had first met, though by French standards still significantly overweight. I had fun describing the different exercises I was experimenting with, kickboxing being the latest.

Since gyms are uncommon and female kickboxers even rarer, the family members looked at me with puzzlement. Were they not familiar with kickboxing, or did I just announce in my broken French, "Last week I tried pig-hopping"?

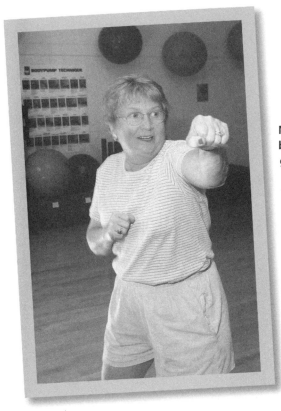

Note to self: Never do kick boxing again! Shopping for groceries on the way home, I almost hoped someone would cut ahead of me in the checkout line so I could demonstrate my new skills. Luckily for me, no one did. The next day I could barely move.

Different Place, Same Commitment

I kept my commitment to fitness in France the same way I did at home—one day, one meal, at a time. When eating in the home of my son's French family, I learned not to finish everything on my plate—it only invited a second helping. I thought they pretended not to notice when I played with my food in order to avoid overeating.

Because so many family members were joining us, my husband and I rented a house outside of Uzes in the middle of a vineyard. Each day I walked for an hour. As I hiked, my eyes were treated to endless vineyards dotted with beautiful gray stone houses with brightly painted shutters. Sometimes my walk was inadvertently extended by a half hour or more when I got disoriented in the vineyards. But what a beautiful place in which to be lost!

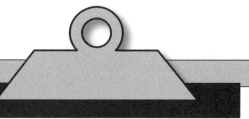

Progress Report
Week 6

Description	Start 7/13	Now 8/21	Goal 11/2	Result to Date
Weekly exercise	2 hrs/wk	7 hrs/wk	12 hrs/wk	Increased 5 hrs/wk
Weight	179	162	139	Lost 17 pounds
Total measurements*	381	351	341	Lost 30 inches

* Total measurements include neck, chest, bust, upper torso, waist, hips, upper thighs, lower thighs, upper arms, lower arms, calves, wrists, ankles.

Progress *Bonjour! Provence est très jolie.* The wine and food, especially the presentation, are extraordinary. At each decision point, I try to make the best, if not the perfect, choice. When I am sorely tempted, my mantra is, "Once on the lips, forever on the hips." I dropped two inches and two pounds this week.

Obstacles I lost two days of exercise to travel. I feel as if I am walking through a minefield of croissants, desserts, cheeses, breads, sausages—any one of which can blow my regimen to bits. It's very difficult to stay focused on my long-term goal. I have no idea if I can stay on track. We'll see.

Why Don't French Women Get Fat?

Self-respect is the fruit of discipline;
the sense of dignity grows with the ability
to say no to oneself.
RABBI ABRAHAM HESCHEL

The law correlating the amount of food consumed and the size of the person seemed to be suspended in France. My French daughter-in-law wore size 2, but only after a big meal. Her mother, approaching fifty, wore size 4.

Moreover, they did not appear to be the exception. Everywhere I went in southern France, I saw trim, slender men and women. I was twice the size of most of them.

In Heaven—Almost

A typical day's eating in the home of my French relatives began with a chocolate croissant, some fruit, yogurt, and coffee or tea, a deceptively simple beginning.

Lunch became more serious. It started with a hot dish of scalloped potatoes with onions and cheese, accompanied by grilled pork tenderloin steaks, garnished with roasted red peppers marinated in olive oil flavored with garlic. All of the food was washed down with copious glasses of rosé wine.

The second course was a green salad lightly dressed in olive oil and balsamic vinegar. The third course consisted of assorted cheeses with baguettes and fruit. Then we were served almond cake, a cream-filled pastry covered with sliced, rum-flavored, sugared almonds.

Finally, to stay awake for the afternoon, we had small-but-strong cups of coffee sweetened with sugar and hunks of chocolate that were slowly melted on the tongue by the hot coffee.

I was in heaven—except for needing to watch closely how much I ate. I assumed that lunch was the big meal of the day, but I was wrong, wrong, wrong. About 9:00 PM, after cocktails with various finger foods— mussels steamed over a grill in a white wine–based broth, eggplant pâté on bread, puff pastries filled with meat, and marinated olives—we began the serious eating.

Small slices of pizza were served on fluffy pastry layered with mustard, creamy white cheese, sliced fresh tomatoes, and black olives. Baked only until the top ingredients melted, the pizza dissolved in the mouth.

Bow-tie pasta surrounded by hunks of fresh, red tomatoes and other vegetables plus a green salad gave color to the table. Our last major course was grilled tuna steaks with a tomato-based, white wine–onion sauce with various herbs and seasonings.

Again the baguettes and cheese. Then we enjoyed ice cream with real whipped cream topping and broken chocolate pieces scattered on top with a cookie buried in each dessert. Each course was washed down with red, rosé, or white wine until we switched to a sweeter wine to accompany dessert.

When we finished after midnight, my petite hosts commended my discipline in limiting my intake, as they delicately continued to munch away.

With all this food, how in the world did they stay so trim?

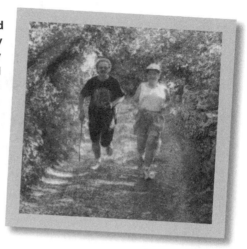

While traveling in France, I needed a photograph to send back to my hometown newspaper for my weekly report. Since trainers are rare, I persuaded my son's French father-in-law to pose as my trainer. A willing accomplice, Jean-Louis suggested we stage the scene—running through the vineyard behind our vacation home. Roxa, his dog, joined us although *le chien* didn't make it into the photo. (The family was disappointed!) My son Steve was the photographer.

"Food Is Life"

Their Mediterranean diet, I noticed, focused on grains, fish, many colorful vegetables and fruits, and olive oil. Adults ate yogurt and cheese but did not drink milk. Except for chocolates and fancy desserts on special occasions, sugar was seldom consumed, except in coffee. The heavier meats, such as beef, were eaten sparingly.

Everywhere, people grew and ate organic food. "Food is life," I heard repeatedly. The good life meant cooking, presenting, and enjoying leisurely meals, accompanied by wine-inspired lively conversation.

As a result, French parents and grandparents frown on the American fast-food restaurants that have invaded the region in recent years. Increasingly popular with the young French, these restaurants are retraining appetites and tastes wholesale. Fast food is also eroding the tradition of enjoying meals with friends and family. Snacking, formerly reserved for small children, is working its way into French eating patterns. All of this was unheard of only a decade ago.

Exercising Regularly

Full-time working people also have time to exercise, since the work week is legendarily short. For example, teachers work twenty-five hours a week with eleven weeks paid vacation plus holidays. Fitness centers

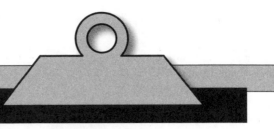

Progress Report

Week 7

Description	Start 7/13	Now 8/31	Goal 11/2	Result to Date
Weekly exercise	2 hrs/wk	8 hrs/wk	12 hrs/wk	Increased 6 hrs/wk
Weight	179	161	139	Lost 18 pounds
Total measurements*	381	350	341	Lost 31 inches

Total measurements include neck, chest, bust, upper torso, waist, hips, upper thighs, lower thighs, upper arms, lower arms, calves, wrists, ankles.

Progress Just maintaining is my definition of progress at this point. I estimate that I'm spending six hours a day at family meals, including breakfast, lunch, and late-night dinners. I've managed to schedule a little exercise—hiking and swimming, even taking to the waves in the Mediterranean Sea. Results for week: one inch and one pound. Whew!

Obstacles I take a small portion of the food I'm served even if I don't intend to eat it. I don't want to offend our hosts, who have worked weeks preparing for the wedding. With extra food on my plate, trying to minimize the amount of food I eat is not an easy task. I love every minute with my son and his French family, so I'm not complaining. Indeed, I can hardly wait for the wedding.

are uncommon except in bigger cities, so people typically take a leisurely walk or go hiking.

The paths and trails were safe and well marked everywhere I went. I hiked every day, hoping to offset the results of heavier eating. I also used the swimming pool at our rented house daily, reveling in the cooling plunge after the hundred-degree heat of midday.

The cuisine, however healthy, was a challenge. Since I would have to choose wisely wherever I went in life, I thought I might as well practice in France. What a delightful challenge!

The Lull
before the Storm

Remember, no matter where you go, there you are.
EARL MACRAUCII

On the day of the wedding, as I had promised myself, I ate whatever I wanted and as much as I wanted. Festivities began with lunch at the bride's home. In an upstairs bedroom a makeup artist worked on the entire bridal party, including this soon-to-be mother-in-law. In the excitement of becoming photogenic, I forgot all about food.

The wedding began with a walk to the mayor's office for a civil ceremony and photographs. Afterward we formed a caravan of cars to the chateau for another ceremony—this one more personal and spiritual. Champagne and hors d'oeuvres followed for guests. After a short break, about a hundred close friends and family members retired to a banquet hall on an estate built in a century past. There we enjoyed a formal dinner complete with entertainers, wine, ceremonies, toasts, a band, and dancing.

Each of the dozen or so courses (too many to keep track of) was accompanied by red and white wines. Interspersed with champagne toasts, we ate our way through the evening until well after midnight and then danced until dawn. Whatever extra calories I consumed were more than made up for by six hours of dancing, an extraordinary feat! By the time I returned to California, I had lost another three pounds and five more inches.

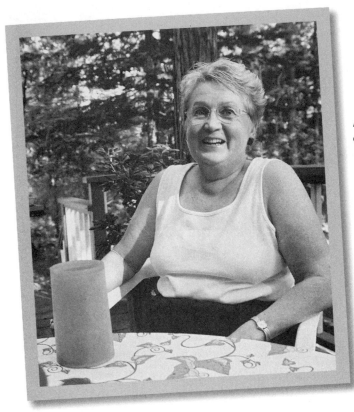

After two weeks of resisting delightful French temptations, I'm relieved to be back at home with access to my own kitchen, surprised that I'm eager to resume my regimen.

Progress Report
Week 8

Description	Start 7/13	Now 9/7	Goal 11/2	Result to Date
Weekly exercise	2 hrs/wk	8 hrs/wk	12 hrs/wk	Increased 6 hrs/wk
Weight	179	158	139	Lost 21 pounds
Total measurements*	381	345	341	Lost 36 inches

Total measurements include neck, chest, bust, upper torso, waist, hips, upper thighs, lower thighs, upper arms, lower arms, calves, wrists, ankles.

Progress Inches drop faster than pounds—over an inch for every pound lost. Inches are now dropping off the torso, especially waist, as my former figure begins to emerge. Oh, happy day! Although I had two "free" eating days—wedding day and groom's dinner—I returned immediately to my regimen: a relief! Even after traveling, amazing results for the week! I look forward to rejoining the tennis clinic—it is a fun way to log exercise hours. Soon I will have to alter my clothes or give them away.

Obstacles While traveling, maintaining an exercise regimen with only myself to listen to was especially difficult. My excuses were remarkably creative. It's a good thing I traveled with my scale—it kept me honest. When choosing food, I wonder if I will always prefer the fattening over the nutritious, the rich over the healthful. Will I always need to be disciplined? I need to take a moment to enjoy the progress I've made.

Everything Changes

Security is mostly a superstition. It does not exist in nature. . . .
Life is either a daring adventure or nothing.

HELEN KELLER

My sister, Kay, who lives in Iowa, called me on September 11 as the events in lower Manhattan were unfolding. I rarely watch daytime television and was unaware of the drama. My husband and I turned on the television only to watch in horror the dramatic footage of two planes crashing into the World Trade Center.

Then our television went blank; our power was out! Were power lines being attacked in California? Without electricity, we huddled around a battery-operated radio, listening for the smallest scrap of news.

Our world seemed to be falling apart. Later we learned that the two events were unrelated; nonetheless, the illusion of invulnerability had been stripped from our reality. Taking life for granted was a luxury we could no longer afford.

Like other Americans, I was shocked by the terrorist attacks. Everywhere, I heard the same words: "Nothing will ever be the same." Like others, for the first time in my life I was fearful of the future.

In the accompanying sadness, I found myself shrinking from my commitment to fitness. Suddenly the effort seemed irrelevant and naive. I wanted to cocoon at home and make the world go away. What difference did my puny efforts make? I stood at a crossroads.

Give Up or Get Going—My Choice

After reflection, I realized that just as I had been challenged in the past, I would be challenged in the days ahead. Facing the future as fit as possible would give me the strength, resiliency, and energy to deal with the needs of my family, friends, and community in uncertain times. Instead of retreating, I'd hang the American flag on our front porch each day and exercise more than ever.

My hero became Erma Ford, a Red Cross volunteer nurse who, at seventy-four, worked on relief efforts at Ground Zero in New York. I didn't know if I would ever have to run from a burning building, rescue a stranger, raise a grandchild, suffer the loss of a family member, or help

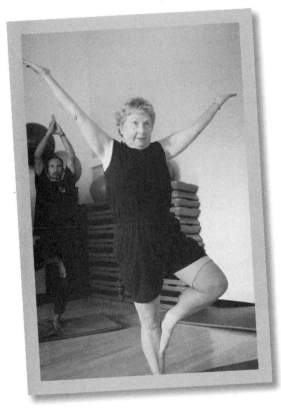

My very first yoga class—an awful sixty minutes. I struggle for balance while my classmate easily maintains the tree pose. Unless Gayle insists, I won't return.

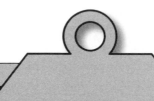

Progress Report
Week 9

Description	Start 7/13	Now 9/14	Goal 11/2	Result to Date
Weekly exercise	2 hrs/wk	12 hrs/wk	12 hrs/wk	Reached goal
Weight	179	155	139	Lost 24 pounds
Total measurements*	381	341	341	Lost 40 inches, reached goal

* Total measurements include neck, chest, bust, upper torso, waist, hips, upper thighs, lower thighs, upper arms, lower arms, calves, wrists, ankles.

Progress Today is a wonderful day to be alive and free. I give thanks for all that is good. I reached my goal in inches! Additional losses will be gravy. Whoops! Wrong word for someone on an eating regimen. Gayle says weight training really trims, although even she's surprised at how quickly I am moving toward my goals. I've also reached my weekly target of twelve-plus exercise hours. Weekly result: I lost three pounds and four inches. I feel alert and emotionally strong, prepared to deal with whatever life offers.

Obstacles Horrific events during the week took their toll. Sadness for families with losses overwhelms me at times. The awareness of the presence of evil is difficult. I could slack off, but I refuse to give the terrorists anything more than what they have already brutally taken. Instead, I recommit.

a teenager who needed a friend, but I wanted to be prepared. Instead of depending on others for daily care or dying prematurely because of a self-indulgent and sedentary lifestyle, I'd become healthy and fit so I could extend that care to others if needed. Instead of retreating, I'd move forward.

Difficulties Ahead

I knew the hardest part might still lie ahead. How could I be confident that having worked so hard to get to this point, I wouldn't slip back into my old ways? Once I had reached my goal weight, how would I maintain it?

Like brushing teeth, choosing to eat healthily and maintain an exercise regimen, day in and day out for the rest of my life, would have to become a nonnegotiable discipline. As world events reminded us, though, living isn't for sissies, is it?

You Gotta Have Friends

We're all in this alone.

LILY TOMLIN

Because Gayle insisted, I returned to the yoga class. The second one wasn't any easier. Poses that others did effortlessly I couldn't do at all. I watched the hands on the clock at the front of the room. Sixty minutes took forever. After the second session, I told the guy behind me that if I had anything to do with it, I wouldn't come back. He smiled, responding that he once had felt the same way. But, just as he was encouraging me to come back, a fellow classmate had urged him to return. Like him, he said, if I returned, I would end up loving that hour.

He was right. Eventually I acquired the habit, and now, several years later, the sixty-minute stretching/yoga routine starts most of my days— and it is my favorite time alone with my body.

Without my classmate's encouragement, I never would have gone back to that yoga class. But return I did, week after week. Slowly I found my flexibility increasing even as my body was aging. Plus, I began to make wonderful new friends, an unexpected and delightful benefit of my fitness project. Now more than halfway into my four months of fitness training, I was finding companions on the journey.

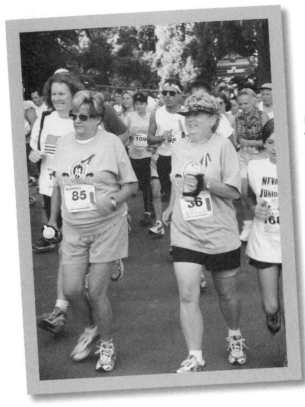

I (on the right) start the 5K Clydesdale Classic run/walk, accompanied by my tennis partner, Dale (left), and her workout partner, Ruth (center).

Companions on the Journey

I could no longer buy groceries, pump gas, or shop in my small town without people coming up to me to talk about their own fitness efforts, or lack of them. Readers who followed my weekly newspaper columns couldn't wait to comment on my progress or share their stories with me. A few said they'd started their own programs.

Trips to town now took an extra hour or two because I wanted to listen to each person's story. I could usually count on talking to two or three people in the grocery store, one or two more as I pumped gas, and a couple more at the bank either going out or coming in. Most greeted me by name, which left me wondering how I knew them.

Once the conversation turned to fat and fitness and pounds, however, I knew the person was just like me—searching to find a way to get fit.

Progress Report
Week 10

Description	Start 7/13	Now 9/21	Goal 11/2	Result to Date
Weekly exercise	2 hrs/wk	14 hrs/wk	12 hrs/wk	Goal + 2 hours
Weight	179	151	139	Lost 28 pounds
Total measurements*	381	336	341	Goal + 5 inches, total 45 inches

* Total measurements include neck, chest, bust, upper torso, waist, hips, upper thighs, lower thighs, upper arms, lower arms, calves, wrists, ankles.

Progress What a joy to talk with readers tracking my progress and setting up their own regimens! Even my tennis coach comments that I am more coordinated now that I carry around less weight. Gym workouts continue to trim, while yoga helps with stretching and flexibility. This week I lost four pounds and five inches. Daily I wear red, white, and blue ribbons to remind me of what others have already sacrificed, as well as sacrifices yet to be made.

Obstacles Competing in the 5K walk/run intimidated me. My eyes sprang open Sunday morning once I remembered I'd signed up for a competitive event in a sport for which I have little talent. My first reaction was to pull the covers over my head and go back to sleep. I told myself no one would notice if I didn't come. I'm glad I didn't chicken out because it was so much fun! In fact, I'm going to sign up for more events! Tough times demand resilience and stamina. Whatever the future holds, I want to be fit.

Sometimes another stranger would overhear our conversation and join in, especially when I was in the fabric store. All of a sudden I would find myself in a circle of women talking and laughing about our efforts to shape up.

In public settings, these strangers made startlingly personal confessions to me and others in our group about overeating and their determination to change. Listening to them, I felt like a minister forgiving the repentant and telling them to go forth and sin no more. I wasn't sure what else to do. Some asked for advice. It was tempting to give, but I wasn't qualified. Other than the general wisdom—"Eat less and exercise more"—I encouraged them to see their doctors, visit a gym, get a health and risk assessment, and take baby steps toward fitness.

That's What Friends Are For

This week I received an invitation to be the honorary guest to begin the 5K and 10K run/walk, the Clydesdale Classic, at the Nevada County Fairgrounds. Since I wasn't a runner, I decided I would begin the race with a light jog and then drop back to walk the remainder. Not wanting to go alone, I persuaded my new friend and tennis partner, Dale, to join me.

Responding to the sound of the starting horn, Dale and I began the race in the cold late-autumn morning air. We jogged until we were safely out of camera range. Talking all the while, we walked as fast as we could—more to keep warm than to compete with other athletes—until we crossed the finish line.

Later, while waiting for friends to pack up, I watched the race organizers report results and hand out medals to winners. Suddenly my ears perked up. Was that my name he just called? Surprise! I had placed second in my age category. I figured only two people had registered in my age group—and the other person took first place. But I certainly enjoyed walking to the stage and receiving my medal, to the accompaniment of applause from onlookers.

What Does It Take?

Everything is connected. . . . No one thing can change by itself.
PAUL HAWKEN

When I started my makeover, Debbie Wagner, coordinator of the Wellness Center at Sierra Nevada Memorial Hospital, offered to add a medical perspective. As part of a "Personal Wellness Profile," I completed a lengthy questionnaire and underwent various tests and measures—flexibility, blood pressure, weight, percent body fat, lung capacity, and so on.

The result was a personalized twenty-page report. Among other red alerts, I was in the ninetieth percentile for risk of heart disease. The risk of cancer was also elevated because of excessive body fat, which amounted to nearly 40 percent of my total body mass.

The physiologist who reviewed the report encouraged me to eat differently and exercise. If I implemented the changes, my physiological age would be a decade or more less than my chronological age. Although the calendar would say I was sixty, my body would perform like that of a fifty-year-old.

Despite this life-critical information, I still found making lifestyle changes tough. There were so many hidden rewards and benefits in the way I had once lived. In the past, I had escaped responsibility for my health by shifting the responsibility to my doctor. And why not? I

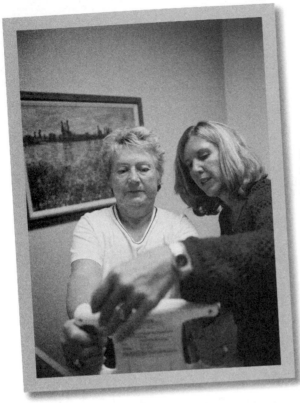

Debbie Wagner, RN, enters numbers into a handheld device that measures the body's fat-to-muscle ratio.

believed that any medical consequences of my self-indulgent lifestyle, if they occurred at all, would happen in the far distant future. Now much older, I wanted to go whole hog—eating and drinking as I pleased.

To further complicate matters, living alongside the hedonist in me was the straitlaced contrarian who believed that I should be sufficiently self-disciplined to make necessary changes. Because I believed I should be strong, it never occurred to me to get help.

No wonder I'd tried and failed in the past!

Now I had help; I had the support of Gayle, my husband, and the countless others who were following my progress in the newspaper. Would I make my goals by my birthday, November 5? I had no idea. But I was enjoying the progress so far. I vowed again not to give up!

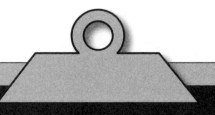

Progress Report
Week 11

Description	Start 7/13	Now 9/28	Goal 11/2	Result to Date
Weekly exercise	2 hrs/wk	16 hrs/wk	12 hrs/wk	Goal + 4 hrs, solid achievement
Weight	179	149	139	Lost 30 pounds —10 left
Total measurements*	381	334	341	Lost 47 inches

* Total measurements include neck, chest, bust, upper torso, waist, hips, upper thighs, lower thighs, upper arms, lower arms, calves, wrists, ankles.

Progress This week I worked out with weights for three hours and per- formed yoga exercises for one and a half hours. Exercise is my "job" until I reach maintenance. Additional hours of tennis are playtime. Sunday is a day for rest. I lost two pounds and two inches this week.

Obstacles Weights and yoga require discipline. Like artichokes and anchovies, they're acquired tastes. Building muscle and bone density, along with increasing flexibility, is as important as aerobic exercise (such as tennis) but not as easy, at least for me. It's a good thing I have a trainer and yoga instructor to keep me on track.

The More I Lose,
the More of "Me" There Is

The one thing nobody can do better than you is be you.
ELIZABETH MOON

Wardrobe changes were in order. My old clothes were too big, but I didn't want to buy new ones until I knew my final size. Consignment stores could keep me clothed until I knew where I'd end up, but I did splurge on new underwear.

The Old Me Beckons

Now a new temptation beckoned. The closer I got to my goal, the more frequently I found myself thinking about abandoning the project. As excited as I was about progress, I was also drawn back to the familiarity of the "old" me. The more my body changed, the stronger this impulse to run away to a "safe" place where I could eat french fries and double bacon cheeseburgers without reproach for my public commitment to fitness.

I felt sad about the person I was leaving behind. One day I actually mourned her, the way you mourn a dear friend who has moved away. In the best way she knew, she had seen me through some tough times. Now I was leaving her to find a new friend.

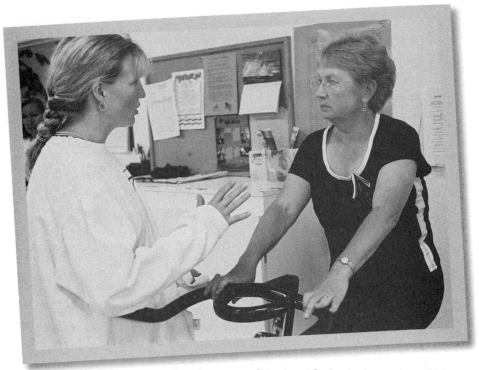

Despite my conditioning, I find spinning an incredible challenge. Hooked up to a heart-rate monitor, I keep a safe pace during the one-hour class taught by Carolyn Hansen. When I finish and dismount the bike, I can barely walk. I think I'll stick with tennis.

Do I sound crazy? Well, that's how I felt. Like a fading photograph, the former "me"—a person of substance—was disappearing. Emerging in her place was the new "me," a petite and feminine woman. This new person was more exposed, more vulnerable, and more available to others. She definitely wanted to come out and play.

Bridging the old and new person was the "me" always present whatever the form, the person who never changed and never would. Sometimes I felt as if I were on a roller coaster, the transition between what-was and what-was-yet-to-be both exhilarating and frightening. However the experiment turned out, though, I was glad I'd had the courage to buy the ticket and take the ride.

Progress Report
Week 12

Description	Start 7/13	Now 10/5	Goal 11/2	Result to Date
Weekly exercise	2 hrs/wk	12 hrs/wk	12 hrs/wk	Reached goal but difficult week
Weight	179	147	139	Lost 32 pounds
Total measurements*	381	331	341	Lost 50 inches

* Total measurements include neck, chest, bust, upper torso, waist, hips, upper thighs, lower thighs, upper arms, lower arms, calves, wrists, ankles.

Progress With worrisome uncertainty still hanging in the air from the September 11 attack, it seems important to get and stay fit, if only for peace of mind. I managed to log twelve exercise hours this week even though three days were spent in the car looking at fall colors around Lake Tahoe. This week I lost two pounds and three inches. Other good news: Gayle was selected by the U.S. Olympic Committee to carry the Olympic torch for Nevada County as it crosses the country.

Obstacles I have to remind myself of the benefits of change. Despite my progress to date, daily I feel the urge to escape by moving away. Whose idea was this to do the newspaper series anyhow? The next moment I'm reenrolled and enjoying the process, especially when strangers tell me they've started their own fitness programs after following my progress.

Entering the Home Stretch

Physical health is not a commodity to be bargained for.
Nor can it be swallowed in the form of drugs and pills.
It has to be earned through sweat.

B. K. S. IYENGAR

Since July, two changes—eating differently and exercising more—had transformed my body. When individuals approached me with their plans, I quickly pointed out that this was the toughest work I'd ever attempted. I also added that between the two changes, exercising was a piece of cake compared to eating differently. (Whoops, wrong analogy!)

Failure Rate Is High

Evidently I wasn't alone. In a free, nationwide health program called "Choose to Move" involving 23,000 women, over 19,000 dropped out. The results of the American Heart Association study, reported in the *Archives of Internal Medicine* on October 8, 2001, show how hard it is to stick with healthy lifestyle changes, even if intentions are good.

The AMA also reports that cardiovascular disease is the number one killer, accounting for 40 percent of all premature deaths—450,000 people annually. High blood pressure is a silent killer, and elevated cholesterol is linked to heart disease and stroke. Moreover, the Centers for Disease Control and Prevention reports that the incidence of diabetes continues to accelerate.

Since the health risks of being overweight are increasingly alarming, why is it so difficult to live a healthy lifestyle?

"Now" Never Seems Like the Right Time

First, "now" is never a good time to begin. "Tomorrow" looks more promising. "Now," in fact, seems like an especially good time to indulge oneself. As far as I can tell, though, the right time to begin does not exist.

Second, dietary changes result in immediate losses before long-term benefits show up. You may have to lose favorite foods or supersized portions before you can lose the pounds. When everyone else indulges, delayed gratification is a tough sell. What a leap of faith!

I've also discovered reasons for eating that have nothing to do with nutrition. In my past reality, comfort, reward, distraction, recreation, and cravings were perfectly acceptable reasons to indulge. Sometimes I ate because the clock said "time" or, alternatively, to keep from getting hungry. I called it preventative eating. Sometimes I ate because the food smelled good or because of thirst and fatigue.

Eating the Right Food for the Right Reasons

Eating for the intrinsic value of food—nutrition and energy—and not for extraneous reasons was a radical shift. Within a daily caloric allowance, I balanced protein, vegetables, fruits, grains, dairy, and plenty of fluids over three light meals and two snacks. Each decision I made about what to consume was governed by what my body needed, not what I wanted. And although cocktails and wine would have been nice once in a while, I couldn't afford to spend the calories, especially when the calories were "empty" ones void of any nutritional value.

If these difficulties weren't enough, I realized I would never be finished. If I succeed today, tomorrow I must fight again. Giving myself one free day a week might help, but temptations would always abound.

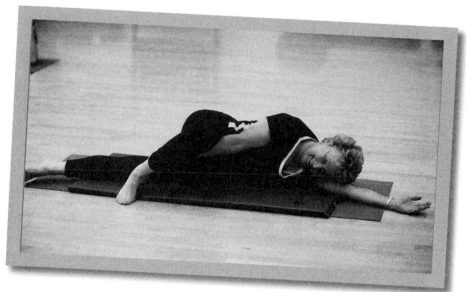

Here I am trying yet another discipline, Pilates, which requires enough bravery to wear tights. What a contrast between the first picture in the newspaper and this one! I can see the new form of my body taking shape. Although Pilates is one of the more challenging exercises I've tried, I enjoy getting down on the floor and "playing" with my body. When I do, I feel like a child again.

I was also ambivalent. The old me—a self-indulgent hedonist—preferred the comfort of elastic waistbands. Habits, food preferences, and unexpected triggers, like the smell of warm cookies fresh from the oven, steered me backward. The new me—the fitness marine—liked the discipline and considered it a patriotic duty to shape up. Ultimately, my body would reflect the "me" who prevailed.

I was amazed at my body's recovery from years of abuse. It wasn't as if my old body just had less weight on it. I felt as if I had a whole new body. The hanging skin folds under my arms were gone, my stomach was flat and hard without extra flab, and my legs looked as they did in high school when I played basketball. If the body isn't miraculous in its functioning, then I don't know what is.

Did I feel and look terrific? Yes. Did I have tons of energy? Yes. Was I sometimes hungry? Yes. Did I miss my treats? Yes. Would I continue? Yes, but only if I found comfort, rewards, and recreation away from the

Progress Report
Week 13

Description	Start 7/13	Now 10/12	Goal 11/2	Result to Date
Weekly exercise	2 hrs/wk	14.5 hrs/wk	12 hrs/wk	Goal + 2.5 hrs, good week!
Weight	179	145	139	Lost 34 pounds —6 left
Total measurements*	381	327	341	Lost 54 inches

Total measurements include neck, chest, bust, upper torso, waist, hips, upper thighs, lower thighs, upper arms, lower arms, calves, wrists, ankles.

Progress I have less inclination to eat inappropriately. New eating habits seem to be the norm—finally! What a joy to move freely in my body and have so much energy! With twenty-one days to go, I'm in the home stretch. Whatever statistics I end up with, I'm thrilled. Approaching sixty next month, I haven't felt and looked this good since college. Why didn't I do this earlier? This week I lost two pounds and four inches.

Obstacles Travel this week makes the eating regimen and exercise difficult, but I need to cope wherever I go. The three hours of Pilates and yoga classes are difficult because I'm not naturally limber. Another three hours of weights in the gym requires similar discipline. My eight hours of tennis is playtime.

dining table; otherwise, I'd put the weight back on. I would also need to remind myself daily of the health benefits and the joy of physical activity without limitations.

Ultimately, though, if I succeeded it would be because when I looked in the spiritual mirror, I liked myself better when I led a disciplined life. It felt good to have a rule—eat consciously for what my body needs—and the discipline to follow it. Permanently, I hoped, self-indulgence had been replaced with a sense of deep privilege for the opportunity to become fit and, by my example, to encourage others to do the same.

On the Road Again

Life is full of obstacle illusions.

GRANT FRAZIER

Having spent his adult life as a family man tied down to his forestry job, my retired husband harbored a pent-up desire for travel that seemed to peak during my fitness efforts. At the risk of sounding paranoid, I wondered if at some level he was testing me to see if he could bring back his party-girl wife! After all, he said, it wasn't nearly as much fun for him to eat and drink alone, especially when I sat across the table from him being so pure and wholesome.

When he proposed a vacation on the Mendocino coast, I had no reason to decline—that is, except for not knowing if I could maintain my regimen while traveling. But after all, I asked myself, what good is a fitness regimen if it won't travel?

I would need a plan of attack. I could take the scale—now my very best friend instead of my enemy—to weigh myself. If we were flying, I could walk briskly during the preboarding time to log a few exercise minutes. But since we were driving, I'd need to get up early and exercise before we left.

Even more worrisome was dining out. My husband likes fancy places with cocktails, tempting entrées, and lovely desserts, and his choice of restaurants in Mendocino would be no exception. While I watched

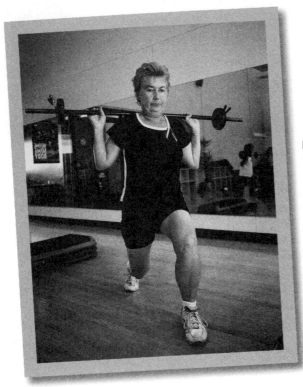

Doing a lunge in a Body Pump class gets the heart rate going, while I wear a red, white, and blue pin in remembrance of September 11.

him enjoy his favorites, I would be forced to remain focused on my own goals.

But I am very stubborn. The more difficult the challenge, the more determined I become. I began thinking about the advantages of eating out and ways I could cope. At least I couldn't walk into the restaurant kitchen and help myself to seconds as I could at home! When ordering, I could get food prepared exactly as I liked, and I could choose what I wanted to eat. I could control portions by ordering appetizers instead of an entrée. I could package food up and take it back to our motel room. And I wouldn't have to spend hours in the kitchen surrounded by temptations.

For exercise, I'd have to be flexible. Because I was keeping up with my classmates in my Body Pump class, I began to think of myself as

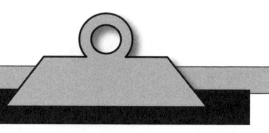

Progress Report
Week 14

Description	Start 7/13	Now 10/19	Goal 11/2	Result to Date
Weekly exercise	2 hrs/wk	16 hrs/wk	12 hrs/wk	Goal + 4 hrs, lots of walking!
Weight	179	144	139	Lost 35 pounds, 5 left
Total measurements*	381	326	341	Lost 55 inches

* Total measurements include neck, chest, bust, upper torso, waist, hips, upper thighs, lower thighs, upper arms, lower arms, calves, wrists, ankles.

Progress   Good news about a prescription drug! My doctor has agreed that the dosage for my beta-blocker will be halved because of my weight loss and exercise; ultimately, I may be able to eliminate it completely. I surprised myself by hiking twenty-one miles in four days. Walking alone on the seacoast while watching waves gave me a lift. I discovered a nearby health club with a tennis court, a pool, a hot tub, a sauna, and a gym for seven dollars a day, a real bargain. I lost one pound and one inch this week.

Obstacles   I learned the hard way to check in with my physician when losing weight. Two hours of weights plus seven hours each of walking and tennis represent a lot of exercise for one week. Even so, final pounds are tough to shed; each one argues to stay.

a jock, a real athlete. I could easily walk three to four miles, more if necessary. I would look for a place to walk along the ocean each day.

Red Alert—Medical Emergency Intervenes

A few days before we left for our trip to the coast, I scared myself and my husband badly. Four months earlier I'd been put on a beta-blocker to silence an unusual heart sound. Although I'd once casually mentioned to my cardiologist that I was losing weight, I hadn't told him how much or over what period of time.

As I was getting ready for bed that night, I passed out cold in the bathroom. I bruised my shoulder and hip on a tile step when I fell. Dick heard the crash. I didn't—I was unconscious from the moment I went down. When I returned to awareness, I tried to get up and walk to the bedroom. I passed out again. I finally crawled on all fours to the bedroom and climbed into bed.

After I passed out again, Dick insisted on taking me to the local emergency room. From my pulse, blood pressure, heart rate, and other tests plus some astute questioning, the emergency room doctor eventually figured out that the beta-blocker prescription was too strong for my current size and weight. Losing weight and exercising had significantly reduced my formerly high blood pressure. Because of the medication, my blood pressure was now too low, and that was why I was passing out.

I had learned a hard and expensive lesson about how important it is to have medical supervision. My doctor needed to be my adviser on my fitness journey. I'd used other resources and collected companions of all sorts along the way—but never thought to include my doctor. Once again I realized that all of us are dependent upon each other for our well-being.

Dick and I left on time for our Mendocino vacation, grateful that the medical emergency was a fading memory.

Nothing Tastes as Good as Being Thinner Feels

Each person must live their life as a model for others.

ROSA PARKS

Throughout those four months, local newspaper readers approached me in the grocery store, in its parking lot, or during my walks. Many of them asked the same questions, and one week before my birthday, I took the opportunity to answer them in my column.

Why did you do this? Where did the idea come from? Out of shape and overweight, I was desperate to get fit for my sixtieth birthday. The birthday present from my cardiologist was a warning about potential heart problems if I did not shape up. My physical condition was poor: I had recently injured myself by exercising without proper conditioning. Thinking that my example could encourage others, I offered to write a single newspaper article for seniors. From there, the idea took on a life of its own.

How did it feel to have your weight, progress, and statistics reported each week? It was not pleasant. Seeing my overweight self in a newspaper photo was shocking and reinforced my commitment. Knowing I'd report my progress each week eliminated the alternative of cheating, although I think I was committed in any event.

How has your husband reacted to your changes? Since this was my project, I didn't expect him to change. Nonetheless, he's been supportive, joining me at the gym and changing his eating patterns.

Why did you get a personal trainer? Without a trainer, I literally didn't know where to begin. I needed someone to organize my exercise efforts and also to hold me accountable and encourage me during tough times. Gayle Lossman did even more—she became a special friend.

Are you stopping now? No. These are, after all, lifestyle changes I'm making. I'll lose eight more pounds to reach my goal, increase my flexibility, and make further health improvements.

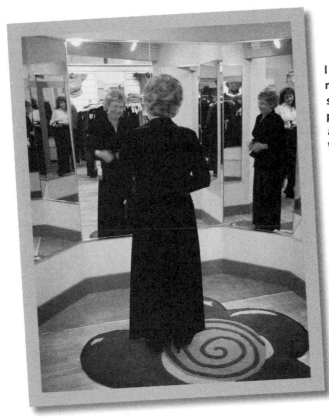

I decided to throw myself a big sixtieth birthday party. That meant a new dress. Wow! I kept trying on smaller and smaller sizes. Finally, a perfect fit! My birthday party dress is four sizes smaller than the size I wore when I started. Am I shocked! I have to get used to the new me.

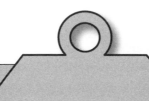

Progress Report
Week 15

Description	Start 7/13	Now 10/26	Goal 11/2	Result to Date
Weekly exercise	2 hrs/wk	12 hrs/wk	12 hrs/wk	Tennis hours are play
Weight	179	142	139	Lost 37 pounds, 3 left
Total measurements*	381	321	341	Lost 60 inches

* Total measurements include neck, chest, bust, upper torso, waist, hips, upper thighs, lower thighs, upper arms, lower arms, calves, wrists, ankles.

Progress   It's hard to believe I have only one week to go! It's been lots of work, fun, and struggle with change during the past four months! When I went shopping, I found that I'm a perfect size 10. Amazing! I'm like a little kid waiting for her birthday party. This week I lost two pounds and five inches.

Obstacles   Losing three pounds in one week to reach my goal seems daunting. I refuse to fast or starve. I won't do anything I can't sustain. Instead, I'll be thrilled with wherever I finish. Exercising regularly and losing seven to nine pounds by New Year's Day is the next goal. Then, a lifetime of maintenance.

Were there any health benefits? My blood pressure went from high to normal, and my resting pulse rate is now in the low forties. The "bad" cholesterol was brought down to normal range, and the "good" cholesterol came way up. I did not have a single sick day. Chronic conditions like gastric reflux and irritable bowel syndrome have disappeared.

What was the hardest part? Giving up a large evening meal was a struggle. Travel posed difficulties because of its association with indulgence. Determination was especially necessary to continue exercising when away from home.

Do you really exercise twelve hours a week? Yes. After experimenting with different exercise disciplines, I settled on working with weights in a fitness center three times a week. I also attend a yoga class to improve flexibility once or twice a week. Lastly, I play tennis, *play* being the operative word.

Could you do this if you had a full-time job and family? Did you consider quitting after September 11? You can't hide behind your obligations to others—your children or your employer, for example—to avoid taking responsibility for the care of your body. You can't find time; you have to make the time. And there is never an easy time to begin. Excuses abound—lack of money and time, medical problems, other priorities. Trust me, I'm familiar with them all because at different times I've used each one of them. Miraculously, a commitment cuts through the obstacles and makes change possible. Ironically, the more fit I am, the more I am able to contribute to my family and employer.

What's the biggest change in your life? Although it's not possible to turn back the hands of time, changing my lifestyle has rewound the clock. An unreasonably optimistic outlook, bountiful energy, a fully engaged life, and a youthful figure are the result of four months of intense work. Until now I never knew results like these were possible, let alone that I would achieve them. That's why I encourage others in as many ways as I can find.

From Shame to Joy

I stand in awe of my body.
HENRY DAVID THOREAU

Although tempted to push the envelope and starve myself to reach my goal, I resisted the impulse and stayed with my ongoing eating and exercise regimen. I ended up meeting my target plus one extra—forty-one pounds lost in all. Despite years of abuse, my body was amazingly responsive. I'd gone from being ashamed to being happy with myself. I was ecstatic at the outcome.

At the same time, I remained fearful that day-to-day life would rob me of momentum and enthusiasm. Would I slip back to my old ways once the exhilaration faded?

Final Report: Success by Any Measure!

Results: Thanks to the miracle of healing combined with strengthening exercises, my hamstring was fine. Exercising daily as well as eating consciously for nutrition and energy were my new norm; the feeling of loss and deprivation was gone. I had lost forty-one pounds and sixty-six inches in sixteen weeks.

Medical tests performed at the beginning and repeated near the conclusion confirmed significant physiological improvements. Blood pressure, resting heart rate, cholesterol, glucose, and body fat were

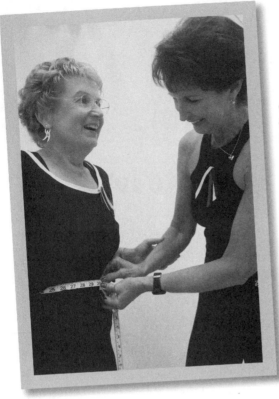

Gayle and I decided that for our last photo, we would repeat the first one. This time we wouldn't hide the number when she measured my waist. In the first photo, my waist measured forty-four inches and my gym clothes were size 18. This time my waist measures thirty-three inches, and I'm wearing a size 10.

significantly lower. Lung function, already good, improved slightly. My formerly high risks of cancer, coronary disease, and osteoporosis were reduced. Although the calendar said I was turning sixty, the test results put my physiological age at forty-seven.

Other changes I'd noticed were reduced sleep requirements (down from ten or twelve hours to seven), a different rising time (5:00 AM instead of 8:00 or 9:00 AM), increased energy, and a more optimistic outlook—which, after September 11, was no small accomplishment. Obviously my body had responded quickly to lifestyle changes, making me wonder how long it had patiently waited.

After splurging at the birthday party, I would resume my effort mainly for health reasons. My risk of heart disease was still unacceptably high, so I needed to reduce body fat by losing more weight before going

Progress Report
Week 16

Description	Start 7/13	Now 11/2	Goal 11/2	Result to Date
Weekly exercise	2 hrs/wk	12 hrs/wk	12 hrs/wk	2 hours a day, Sunday is rest
Weight	179	138	139	Lost 4 pounds, total 41
Total measurements*	381	315	341	Lost 6 inches, total 66

* Total measurements include neck, chest, bust, upper torso, waist, hips, upper thighs, lower thighs, upper arms, lower arms, calves, wrists, ankles.

Progress I am thrilled at my progress. Since I am in the mode of losing weight (the regimen no longer feels burdensome), I've decided to go further. I want to realize a lifelong dream—I want to reach a weight of 122 to 125 pounds. I also want to keep sharing the journey through writing. I feel compelled to share the joy of feeling well, fit, and energetic—an experience that I'd denied myself for forty years.

Obstacles Getting to this level of fitness is the toughest job I've ever done, and going back to my old ways is the biggest danger. Letting the results slip away would be disastrous. Besides feeling better about myself, I feel comfortable with my reinvented body and have a new sense of stewardship for its care. Given the wonderful results, I wonder why I didn't do this sooner.

into a maintenance mode. My schedule of exercising six days a week with Sunday off for rest would continue.

To keep myself on track while simultaneously encouraging others to live more healthfully and joyfully, I offered to write a monthly column for the *Union*. The commentary would provide me an opportunity to explore and share the pitfalls of maintaining my new lifestyle. (I was well aware that getting fit and staying fit were two different processes.) The *Union* accepted my offer.

The stories that I'd shared during my sixteen-week makeover plus the accompanying photographs made many readers feel as if they personally knew me. Seniors, working professionals, teenagers, stay-at-home moms, and individuals with injuries or handicaps—many people, it seemed—were thinking about making healthier choices for themselves. After reading about my transformation, they had come to realize they could do the same thing; they were beginning their own journeys.

Their stories intrigued me. Aha! A light bulb switched on. Besides writing about my own efforts, I could tell the stories of others making lifestyle changes. Then even more readers would expand their notions of what was possible.

Like me, these individuals were not fanatics or health-care professionals. They were ordinary people who had come to realize that their unhealthy lifestyles were making them fat and/or sick. Even if they were illness-free, they realized that the quality of their later years would be negatively affected and perhaps shortened if they didn't change. We were part of an emerging movement—ordinary people struggling to take responsibility for our health and the quality of our lives.

Using my example, they were willing to go public and let me give voice to their stories so that others would be inspired to make healthier life-changing choices.

Although we didn't know it at the time, we were sowing the seeds for a much larger effort.

PART 2

Learning as I Go—
Continuing the Journey

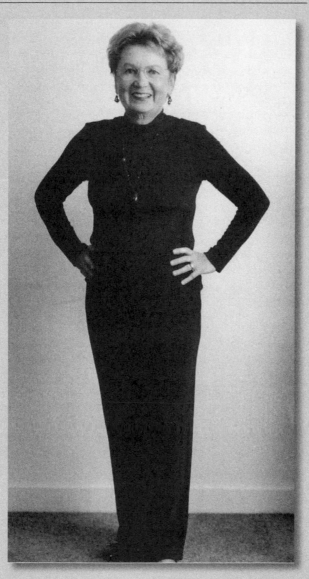

Follow the grain in your own wood.

HOWARD THURMAN

) (

Ecstatic at having achieved the goal set for my sixtieth birthday, I decided to continue my journey. Having a photograph of myself 16 weeks later weighing 138 pounds was joyful, but I wanted to go further. Over the next two months, I lost another twenty pounds, eventually reaching the new me of 122 to 125 pounds, easily fitting into a size 6.

Along the way I altered or gave away my "fat" clothes. Saying good-bye to some of my favorite outfits was hard, but I knew that if I kept them I would be tempted to grow back into them. With only current-sized clothes in the closet, I couldn't go into denial if I started to put pounds back on. Also important was changing my self-image. Every morning when I looked in the closet, I wanted my wardrobe to reflect that I was indeed a fit person.

Once I felt reasonably certain of my new shape, I splurged on new clothes. With the help of a friend who agreed to be my personal shopper, I went to the San Francisco Bay Area to an upscale consignment store. Two hours later I'd purchased a salmon-colored silk Escada pantsuit, a dramatic black-and-white Versace suit, and a beautiful red Valentino sweater all in size 6. Because the clothes were secondhand, the total cost barely reached $150—a real bargain.

Arriving home, I skipped into the house to show my husband the new clothes. "If anyone had ever told me I'd be wearing a Versace suit in size 6, I'd have thought they were doing some serious drugs!" I laughed.

My only regret was that I hadn't made these changes earlier. How could I resist spreading the good news to others? I wanted those I cared about to share the health and emotional benefits that I now enjoyed. I had become a fitness evangelical.

) (

Am I Crazy Enough to Think I Can Change the World?

I'm an idealist. I don't know where I am going,
but I'm on my way.

CARL SANDBURG

Through my continuing monthly column in the *Union*, I encouraged readers on their own journeys by spotlighting the stories of neighbors and friends taking creative routes to fitness.

One of the first people I talked with was Mimi Malthan, a martial arts teacher. During my own makeover, one form of exercise I'd neglected to explore was the martial arts. Curious about what was available, I scanned the yellow pages, found a local studio, and called. The enthusiastic owner suggested I talk with his star pupil. Mimi, he assured me, would inspire me as she had so many others. He wasn't kidding. When I interviewed Mimi, I realized that the long life strides of this seventy-one-year-old made my progress look like baby steps.

Do "Youthing" Instead of Aging—It's More Fun!

"Write your own story with your life," Mimi Malthan tells her students at Mountain Wind Dojo. She encourages them to challenge themselves with the unconventional. "Who says you must behave a particular way at

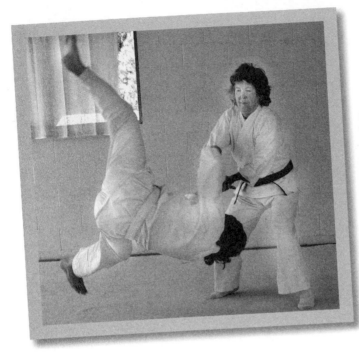

Mimi Malthan, 71, aikido black belt, throws her grandson Chip Currie, 15, at Mountain Wind Dojo in Nevada City.

a certain age?" she asks. "Don't believe the myths you hear about aging. Consider 'youthing' instead. Make your own rules, remembering that the power of your mind is awesome."

Mimi walks her talk. She holds a black belt in Aikido and also an honorary black belt in Sambo, a more aggressive martial art than Aikido.

Mimi's Joy: Making a Difference in Others' Lives

Mimi had a tough time picking her favorite achievement. Along with earning an master of science degree in psychology, raising twenty-seven foster sons was high on the list. Regarding her physical accomplishments, she was especially enthusiastic in describing a three-month-long hike along the Appalachian Trail. In her sixties at the time, she hiked thirteen miles a day carrying a forty-pound backpack.

"It was the most difficult thing I've ever done—and the most rewarding," she said. "Out there on the trail, it's just you and yourself.

Communication with the Spirit is unbelievable. I would do it again in a minute." And why not? She's only seventy-one.

Mimi attributes her good health to her careful eating regimen plus a lifetime of regular exercise. Her extended family, including daughter Asia Currie and grandson Chip Currie, shares Mimi's enthusiasm for martial arts.

I interviewed Mimi but never had the courage to try martial arts. When I sent my visiting granddaughters to her class, they came back in shock over being thrown to a mat by someone a lot older than their grandmother. Both asserted that they would no longer trust people with gray hair!

Fitness Evangelist

Given my role as fitness evangelist, I began proselytizing everywhere. Even my recalcitrant husband was moving toward fitness. He was playing tennis more regularly, had added a flexibility class to his routine, and was being more selective about eating. My older son, Marc, whose cholesterol was unreasonably high, had started talking about changes he could make. My younger son, Steve, also with high cholesterol, started dropping pounds. Could one person make a difference?

I marveled at what was happening around me. Here I thought I was making changes for myself. I never realized that once I changed, the people around me would start changing as well. We seem to be connected in ways we may not fully understand. Being contagious doesn't have to be a problem; it can be healthy, too!

That delightful insight, however, carried with it a responsibility. If I wanted to lift others up, as Mimi was doing, I needed a foundation, the kind that comes from living true to my own standards. That meant maintaining my fitness regimen. The example I set would always speak louder than any words. Well aware of my shortcomings—and even now worried about backsliding—I wished I could pass responsibility for leadership to someone more qualified.

Still, my heart was drawn to this self-imposed task. To quiet self-doubt and anxiety, I reassured myself that I didn't have to succeed—all

I had to do was try. That notion lightened the load; I surrendered to my fitness ministry.

And in the space created by surrender, all sorts of ideas and plans began to percolate. I didn't know where my efforts would take me, or even whether they would be useful to others, but I was on the move.

No matter what tasks I undertook, though, I promised myself that my first priority would remain my own fitness and well-being.

) (

Suffering First-Degree Burns
While Carrying the Torch of Fitness

*No one can listen to your body for you. . . .To grow and heal,
you have to take responsibility for listening to it yourself.*

JON KABAT-ZINN

Opening my eyes, I found myself disoriented by a view of San Francisco Bay in the distance. It took a few seconds before I remembered where I was. The night before, my husband and I had made an unscheduled emergency car trip to Alta Bates Medical Center in Berkeley. Desperately miserable during the four-hour drive, I had felt chest pain so intense that at times I'd resorted to breathing techniques I'd used decades before, during labor.

For the past seven years I'd been having recurring episodes of chest pain accompanied by loud heart sounds, sort of like knocking on wood and easily audible to anyone standing next to me. Repeated trips to the local emergency room and cardiologists' exams had assured me I wasn't having heart attacks. So what was going on? Why were the attacks becoming more frequent and intense?

In addition to chest pain, I'd also suffered a ministroke a few weeks earlier, probably from pushing myself too hard on a run. The numbness in my left arm and the distortion of my face receded in about a week, but the episode worried me because I knew it raised my risk for another stroke. I couldn't eliminate the risk, but I vowed never again to exercise so hard that I couldn't talk at the same time—a prudent, if somewhat tardy, step.

I'd kept my weight stable for three months but could feel my strength slipping away. I noticed that during my time in the emergency rooms, being hooked up to oxygen gave me relief from the chest pain. But once home, the pain would return. My older son, Marc, concerned about my health, came home and arranged for me to get a prescription for oxygen. As each day passed, I could do less and less. I had become an invalid, sitting in my chair, tethered to my oxygen tank. I was desperate for answers. When the pain reached the point that even oxygen would not take it away, my husband and son arranged for me to be admitted to Alta Bates, where comprehensive tests could be run by a team of specialists.

I would spend the next eight days in critical care in the most distress I'd felt since giving birth to my children.

At Last—a Diagnosis!

The team finally identified the problem: esophageal spasms. A calcium channel blocker was prescribed, and treatment began. The pain and sound slowly receded, and I eagerly left the hospital. Thrilled to have found a solution to my medical nightmare, I couldn't wait to resume normal life.

On my first day home, I arose before dawn and went downstairs to fix breakfast, delighted to be returning to my usual routine. However, I needed the railing to steady myself as I went downstairs—that was new. I opened the refrigerator door and realized I was too weak to stand long enough to prepare a bowl of cereal and milk.

Discouraged and disappointed, I retreated to a sofa chair in the living room. Too fatigued to move, I watched as sunlight, seemingly summoned by the singing of birds, took over the sky. While picking away at a sewing project on my lap, I waited for my husband to wake and reflected on the assumptions I'd made about fitness.

Fitness Is No Guarantee

I thought about the hours I'd spent exercising to recover a high level of fitness. Once I'd become fit my medical problems would disappear, right? Fitness was my insurance policy against the impermanence of life! Others might trust financial security, but my confidence derived from knowing that I had shaped up and was living a "pure" life.

I ate carefully, managed my weight at 122 pounds, exercised regularly, eliminated caffeine, and took vitamins and minerals. Because of these efforts my "bad" cholesterol was low, along with my blood pressure.

So why was I unable to perform even the smallest physical task? Why was I now unable to function as I had before? My medical condition wasn't life threatening but it surely was lifestyle threatening!

Reality has a way of teaching even the most stubborn of students. Sitting alone as the sun rose, I let the lesson sink in: fitness wasn't a coat of armor that could fend off the slings and arrows of misfortune. Instead, it was a box of tools that would help me deal more effectively with the uncertainties of life.

Fitness wouldn't prevent all medical problems, but it could help me recover faster.

Did Weight Loss Trigger the Crisis?

I asked various doctors if weight loss or exercise triggered the problem, even though I knew the chest pain had started well before my fitness regimen. I wondered whether I had suffered first-degree burns while carrying the torch of fitness.

On the contrary, as more than one physician told me, my recent weight loss and fitness efforts were my strengths. My timing had been perfect. Facing a medical crisis while I was sixty pounds overweight and had high blood pressure would not have been good. Being strong helped me get through tests, drugs, and intrusive procedures with a minimum of trauma, and it probably also minimized the effects of the transient stroke.

Most happily, I had no future restrictions. After five weeks of deconditioning plus hospitalization, I would need a month to get back to full strength. I vowed never again to take my health for granted.

A *UFO* Strikes—Another "Unexpected Fitness Obstacle"

Four weeks later, eager to resume my fitness efforts, I went for a hike on a nearby trail. The running path was littered with rocks and tree roots. As I alternately ran and walked, I carefully monitored my chest pain. To my delight, I felt none. But wouldn't you know it? I tripped on a root and took a spill, falling face forward with my left leg twisted underneath me.

Face flat on the ground, I started crying—not because of the pain in my leg, which was considerable, but because I knew that I had once again torn a tendon in a hamstring, this time in the other leg. Experience told me the injury meant weeks if not months of recovery. This fitness "thing" was just too darn hard! What was I going to do? It was now my turn to seek courage from what other people had accomplished.

I didn't have to look far.

Never Too Late to Compete

One woman, Susan Michalski, inspired me with her late-in-life accomplishments and the incredible discipline it took to acquire her weightlifting skills. When I met her at the gym and heard her story, I immediately identified with her because I had also been a single parent and typically worked several jobs. Unlike Susan, though, until I retired I didn't have the energy to add a fitness makeover to my to-do list. Nor did I have the imagination to even dream about becoming a competitive athlete.

Raising three kids while working full time at several jobs, Susan didn't find it easy to squeeze in visits to the gym. Only by making it a priority (waking at 3:00 AM and working out until 6:00 AM) was Susan able to succeed beyond her wildest dreams.

After joining a women's power-lifting team at fifty-five years old, Susan set three world records, in squat, dead lift, and bench press, and won state and regional awards in Nevada and California.

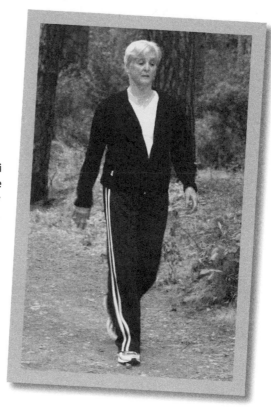

Susan Michalski
demonstrates the
skills that made her
a champion.

Instead of entering her elder years feeling fat and disappointed with herself (she had been a member of Weight Watchers for twelve years), Susan emerged confident with solid self-esteem.

Now sixty-five, Susan does cardio exercises, body sculpting, Pilates, yoga, and weightlifting. She also walks daily and has become an avid snow skier and hiker. As a printmaker and working artist, Susan says she has "creatively responded to her body and its needs" and enjoys being an example to others.

Would that we all responded to our bodies' needs! Certainly I was a little late picking up the cues from my body; late, however, is better than never. With Susan's example, though, I reassured myself that I could maintain my life of fitness. She also inspired me to join a United States Tennis Association team and begin my own career as a competitive athlete.

) (

Wrestling with Devils

What other dungeon is so dark as one's own heart!
What jailer so inexorable as one's self!

NATHANIEL HAWTHORNE

My childhood nickname was "Francis," as in *Francis, the Talking Mule*, a movie from the fifties. Even then, I'd been known for my stubbornness. During this yearlong fitness journey—or ordeal, as some might more accurately put it—my obstinacy had served me well.

That bullheadedness, along with the medication, had helped me achieve a speedy recovery from the esophageal spasms. It also kept me returning to tennis clinics to improve my game, even though my improvements were modest and probably evident only to the coach.

But at no point was my resolve tested more than in the two months that followed my recovery. Wrestling with temptations daily, I needed every bit of willfulness I could muster.

Demons Arrive Unexpectedly

Three changes unleashed the demons. First, houseguests arrived for extended visits, resulting in palate-pleasing menus, dinners later and bigger than usual, plus many fancy desserts. I was responsible for three meals a day for a group, which kept me completely preoccupied with food—planning, shopping, and preparing. With unlimited opportunities to indulge, I was challenged to stay focused.

Even worse, my exercise schedule disappeared. Gym equipment that earlier screamed, "Exercise here!" turned unexpectedly silent. Instead, clothes, appliances, and furniture yelled, "Launder me!" "Dust me!" and "Vacuum me!" Instead of exercising, I responded to the immediacy of their chorus—all in the name of being a good hostess.

I quickly shifted focus from my own needs to those of others. I stayed up late to talk with my guests and got up early to fix their breakfast, skimping on my own rest. I was thoroughly enjoying my company, but it was distressing to watch my new health habits melt away.

The second set of temptations arose from travel. Needing a break from houseguests, my husband and I, as soon as they left, drove over to the coast for five days of vacation. On this trip I was nearly done in by the irregular eating hours. I would get too hungry and then overeat. I succumbed to my love of recreational eating—dinner out with wine, appetizers, and desserts. Eating late before retiring wasn't a good idea, either. Exercise was a catch-as-catch-can proposition: I often didn't work off my favorite breakfast of eggs, bacon, and hash browns.

Not Easy on the Road

When I finally remembered my vision and returned to my regimen, I encountered unexpected obstacles. Breakfast at the motel didn't seem like a good option. The choices were sugared and oil-rich muffins, fruit juice with added sugar and no fiber, and coffee with caffeine. When I ordered an egg-whites-only omelet, a cup of fruit, and dry toast, only the toast was available. Watching my husband eat his 1,500-calorie breakfast while I nibbled on dry toast was difficult, to say the least.

Eating healthy at the restaurants in the small coastal tourist town was no easier. Choices were limited. For example, fruit was seldom available, but french fries were always on the menu. In addition, meal portions were often supersized. My lack of planning—I could have brought healthy snacks—compounded the problem.

No wonder so few people succeed in keeping weight off! After reaching my goal, I needed more determination rather than less.

Back in the Fat Lane Again!

When I returned home, the days of self-indulgence continued, often culminating in decadent dinners (sometimes with not one but three desserts) followed always by a sense of failure. I felt helpless as the numbers climbed in almost perfect two-pound increments: 122, 124, 126, and higher. At this rate, in six months I would gain back everything I had lost. Would I even stop there? Was all my work for naught?

The turning point came when I awoke in despair one morning at 3:00 AM. In the silence of the sleeping house, I faced my self-defeating behavior. My morale was at its lowest, little more than a puddle on the floor. Desperate for relief, I prayed for help. In that instant I realized that if I wanted to recapture my freedom, I'd have to arm wrestle each personal devil to the ground.

To Err Is Human

I spent the next hour reassuring myself that all was not lost, that I needed to be both patient and compassionate. Condemnation, self-judgment, and blame were counterproductive. I was human. To be human is to make mistakes. Moreover, getting fit involves learning, and learning can be painful! In this situation the best I could do would be to view each fall off the horse as an opportunity to make corrections quickly and joyfully.

I also noticed—and felt reassured by it—that I couldn't violate my eating and exercise standards without major distress. The "rules" were internalized now. This was great news! To live peaceably with myself, I'd have to follow my self-imposed regimen. When I didn't, the emotional discomfort was so great that I would voluntarily return to the straight and narrow. Temptations would never go away, but personal demons could be overcome. Next time I wouldn't underestimate them.

Where the Mind Goes, the Body Follows

At the end of the month, I was back to my former weight of 122 to 124 pounds. I even had a plan for our next car trip. I'd use restaurant dining to my advantage. I could order low-calorie food while my spouse ate what he liked. I would substitute vegetables for french fries or tell the server to leave them off my plate. I wouldn't be tempted by second helpings; there are none in restaurants.

To combat supersized portions, when appropriate I would have half the meal put in a to-go box before I started eating, or I'd simply leave it behind. Wasting food went against my grain, but overconsuming was even more offensive. It was better to leave it in the trash than on my hips. Instead of fighting the system, I'd use it.

Thanks to acupuncture, my hamstring was now 90 percent healed, which meant that I'd be able to exercise on the road. I planned on using motel exercise equipment, swimming in a pool when available, and walking an hour a day. I'd also take along my weights so I could do flexibility and strength-building exercises every morning before we started out. When we visited parks, I'd head out for a brisk hike.

How I wish I had not taken such a difficult and painful detour! At the same time, I wouldn't trade the learning for anything. "Francis" was back in charge.

An Even More Determined Woman

Speaking of willfulness, who could match Peggy Davidson? Gayle Lossman, my trainer, told me about Peggy. Like Gayle, Peggy was active in the local running club. But unlike the other athletes, Peggy was a Johnny-come-lately. She was a heavy smoker at age forty. Then, six years later, she was running hundred-mile endurance events. Wow!

At forty-six, Peggy has completed a hundred-mile endurance run three times. In her latest attempt, beginning in the High Sierra at Squaw Valley, Peggy finished in the foothills at Auburn High School twenty-eight hours later. Her husband, Greg, supported her along the way, providing food, drink, and encouragement.

Six years ago, a more unlikely competitor could not have been found. Heavy smoking had left Peggy so short of breath she couldn't blow out birthday candles. Moreover, she had no experience with sports.

Invited on a hike by acquaintances, Peggy said she found herself hopelessly out of shape. A friend suggested running on a local track to prepare for hiking. Peggy couldn't complete a single lap the first day. Yet

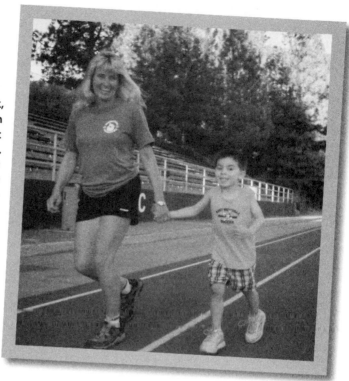

At the local track, Peggy Davidson leads a student in running. Once sedentary and a heavy smoker, Peggy now coaches a running program for kids.

she didn't give up. She volunteered at a local endurance run and there saw participants of all ages, sizes, and shapes. "If they can do it," Peggy thought to herself, "I can do it."

Transitioning in only six years from couch potato to competitive endurance runner required support and discipline. It's a discipline she maintains now that she's met her initial goals. Weekdays at 5:00 AM, Davidson runs for one hour. Weekends she does one or two long-distance runs.

Squeezing in training time isn't easy given her other responsibilities. Peggy is raising two grandchildren, ages six and eleven, while working full time.

Running isn't a chore, Peggy says. Instead, it reduces her stress. Plus, she says, "I feel good about myself—when I'm on the trail and when I finish." Peggy is convinced, "Anyone can run if they set their mind to it."

I'm not sure she convinced me, but, all the same, her achievement is impressive. Perhaps even more impressive, though, is her commitment to coaching kids. Despite everything else on her platter—job, grandchildren, husband, her own training—Peggy finds time to coach youngsters in the sport of running. She's an active member of the Sierra Trailblazers Club, a group of running enthusiasts who share their joy of moving with children.

Most of us will never be able to compete at Peggy's level, but we still can reach out to others, especially children, and share our knowledge and experience. If, through our encouragement, a child learns to enjoy exercise, we all benefit. Thank goodness for exercise angels like Peggy!

) (

Relearning the Three Rs

The time you enjoy wasting is not wasted time.
BERTRAND RUSSELL

If you're a couch potato, you're already a master of "rest," and you can skip this chapter. What follows is written for the "rest-less," those of us who keep going and neglect the body's need for renewal.

When it comes to operating, I have two modes—vertical at full speed or horizontal, too sick or tired to move. I associate rest with something forced on children against their will in the middle of the afternoon. Resting has always seemed like a waste of valuable time. Or is this another idea I need to change?

When Is Enough More Than Enough?

My parents, both farmers in Iowa, were extremely hard workers—a trait that I and my siblings inherited. In my working life, employers appreciated my workaholism. As a single parent, I struggled to get my household tasks done before falling asleep. Now aging, I have an increasingly urgent sense of time running out, so I try to cram as much as possible into each day.

Perhaps this is a common pattern, especially among fitness devotees. The literature of the fitness industry seems to indicate this. Searching for articles on the subject of rest and recovery, I could find only articles focusing on activity. On June 18, 2002, the American Council on Exercise announced the results of a survey of three thousand fitness professionals, which illustrate my point. Asked to name the most common fitness mistakes, the pros listed not warming up adequately, working out too intensely or not intensely enough, not staying hydrated, and eating unneeded high-calorie energy bars. I could name two things they neglected to mention: failing to begin the exercise in a rested body and failing to allow a recovery period.

What I have discovered the hard way is that exercising while fatigued leads to increased risk of injury. This simple point has an important psychological impact for us "rest-less" types. By pushing our bodies to exercise without proper rest, we sabotage our long-term goals to stay fit.

When we're sick, common sense tells us the body heals better and faster with rest. Moreover, new parents don't need researchers to tell them that sleep deprivation does strange things to us. Without enough sleep, I get depressed, anxious, irritable, and depressed. Research also shows that sleep deprivation elevates cholesterol levels. Yet how many of us consider adequate rest an essential part of a long-term fitness regimen?

Work and Rest: Both Are Essential

I finally ratcheted up my courage and signed up to play on an official United States Tennis Association Team. Although it might seem like a small step for some people, for me it was a giant leap. By joining a team, I was making a public statement that I couldn't retreat from. Once on a team, I felt pressure to improve my game so I wouldn't let the team down. I began working extra hard to improve my consistency.

One of my tennis coaches, Greg Cicatelli, noticed that I was struggling with my game and asked me about my schedule. I think he suspected that I was working too hard without giving my body the rest it needed.

When I told him my routine, his normally easygoing manner became stern. He made his point. After my second hamstring tear in a year—the most recent one after I was fit—he warned me to go easier on myself and get more rest. I wondered at first what he was talking about. Now that I was healthy and strong, I felt better than I had at any time since my twenties. I'd proved that my energy was renewable, right?

Renewable, yes, he said, provided I gave it the chance. That meant taking time to rest so my body could do exactly what it was meant to do—recover through rest.

But the notion that "less is more" was counterintuitive to me. With my love for tennis, I was eager to improve. My logic seemed infallible: if two hours of practice six days a week would help me improve, then three a day would take me even further. Yet on this schedule, my game deteriorated. I made mental mistakes and my form broke down.

So what did I do? I practiced more, and my game went even further south. Not allowing adequate recovery time was causing muscle breakdown, lowering future performance. Injuries were more likely.

How ironic, I reflected, that doing nothing—resting—achieves more than continuous effort!

But after his stern lecture, Greg convinced me to take rest and recovery as seriously as I took exercise. He also urged me to stay in touch with my body so I would notice when I was beginning to tire—and quit before I did myself in with an injury. Exercise alone did not improve my body's health and fitness. Instead, health improvements associated with exercise came after I'd finished and allowed my body the proper amount of rest and nutrition.

Restoring Perspective

I also noticed that the psychological benefits of rest were as important as the physiological ones. When I allowed myself to rest, I restored not just my muscles and immune system but also my spirit. Instead of "having" to play tennis, I was looking forward to it again. I've since learned that unexpected, unprogrammed improvements frequently occur after the recovery phase following intense exercise, a delightful benefit of doing nothing.

No doubt I'm the kind of person who should add *rest* to her daily to-do list. While I'm at it, maybe I need to create a not-to-do list to avoid overcommitment. Finally the lesson sank in: taking time to rest has a rightful place in every sustainable fitness regimen.

The Tortoise and the Hare

If I was the hare who rushed out at the start of the race only to fall over in exhaustion before reaching the finish line, Fred Hillerman was the tortoise who kept a steady lifelong pace. How else could you reach eighty-eight and still be moving gracefully forward? And creating a special routine for each day of the week, too!

For some of us, just living that long makes every day special. For years, though, Fred has lived every day of his life that way. I'd heard about this remarkable man through a mutual friend, so I called him to talk.

Fred is retired from two careers—first as a teacher, then as a grower of orchids from Africa and Madagascar. Despite his age, he says he enjoys abundant energy and good health. He feels his life is a walking advertisement for the value of exercise.

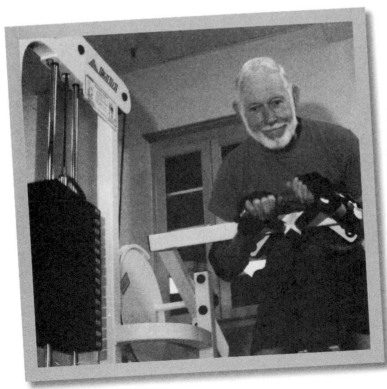

Fred Hillerman, age 88, works out during his regular routine at the local gym.

In addition to serving on the board of directors for the senior center, Fred says he delivers hot food for the Meals on Wheels program. Because he has a regular route, the recipients have become his friends, and Fred keeps an eye on each of them. In addition, one day a week Fred teaches English to Mexican students. The Interfaith Food Ministry also benefits from his volunteer efforts.

Fred hastens to add, though, that his volunteer activities must fit into his exercise schedule. Five or six times a week he lifts free weights at the gym. He's particularly pleased that he can do ten pull-ups.

Besides lifting free weights, Fred takes a spinning class on Mondays, Tuesdays he goes to yoga, and Thursdays he hikes for five to seven hours with the German-American Hiking Club.

Talking to Fred was like talking to an eighty-eight-year-old master of the steady, stable life. Like Fred, I want to live each day with zest as I age. Besides inspiring me, he underscored the benefits of balance and pacing whatever our age. What a joyful person!

) (

A Matter of Life and Death

Do what you can, with what you have, where you are.

THEODORE ROOSEVELT

Just when I thought I'd finally learned all the lessons I needed to learn for a while, I had the rug pulled out from under me.

One Tuesday evening in December, the phone rang as my husband and I were finishing dinner. My granddaughter in Columbia, Missouri, reported that her mother, my thirty-eight-year-old daughter, Jamie, had fainted and was hospitalized. After I absorbed the news, my son-in-law got on the phone and provided more detail.

Jamie had suffered cardiac arrest while checking out of a hotel on a business trip in Oklahoma. A hotel clerk administered CPR until the 911 paramedics arrived and restarted her heart with repeated defibrillations. The time between when her heart stopped and restarted had been dangerously long. She was unconscious when taken by ambulance to a local hospital, where she was stabilized before being moved to a level-one trauma center in Tulsa.

Her husband and three daughters (ages eleven, thirteen, and eighteen) drove the six long hours from their home to the hospital.

I decided to fly to Oklahoma immediately, uncertain what I could contribute but certain I needed to be there. After a sleepless night I left Sacramento in the predawn. Arriving in Tulsa by early evening, I took a taxi to a hotel and checked in, leaving my bags at the front desk so I could head immediately to the adjacent hospital.

Seeing Jamie for the first time was a shock. She was hooked up to countless machines and gadgets, lying still in a coma. Doctors gave her little chance to live.

I huddled with other family members in the intensive care waiting room. Every two hours we were allowed twenty minutes in her room. Over the next two days of our vigil, Jamie gradually regained consciousness, communicating first with her eyes, then in whispers. But as consciousness increased, she became more and more agitated and had to be restrained.

Watching her arms and legs flail and her head roll from side to side was painful and distressing. My fear that she would die was eclipsed by the fear that she'd live and be mentally impaired.

During short breaks I took my granddaughters Christmas shopping, and we had our nails manicured. Sometimes we played cribbage—anything to distract us from the tension of the hospital scene and worrying about what tomorrow might hold.

By Saturday, the third day since her admittance, Jamie had made dramatic progress and was moved to another floor. Unable to care for herself or even ring for help, she couldn't be left alone. Her husband and I traded off feeding her and caring for her basic needs. Eight days after the incident, Jamie was moved to a rehabilitation hospital near her home in Columbia.

During this anxious time, I did try to take care of myself. Although I slept only a couple of hours a night, I ate carefully, albeit irregularly. I walked the hospital corridors, partly for exercise and partly so I could cry privately.

I was strong for those eight days, but by the time I returned home to California, I was a basket case. One moment I was thrilled Jamie had survived. Another moment I'd weep. I felt disoriented and disconnected.

Extra rest and exercise (especially stretching), regular eating, prayers of family and friends, visits to the physical therapist, and especially loving care from a supportive husband restored me. A month later I headed back to Missouri to help Jamie make the transition to home. She could feed and clothe herself, walk with assistance, and communicate, although her short-term memory was still impaired. We hoped she'd recover even though doctors discouraged us from expecting too much from her.

Without being in shape, I would not have survived the trauma nearly as well, nor would I have had the resiliency to return to Missouri and help care for my adult daughter. I was learning another reason to get and stay fit. Until now, I'd shallowly wanted to avoid medical problems, play tennis, and enjoy abundant energy. Silly me! I was preparing for a much greater task, caring for a loved one. I needed to be strong, healthy, and balanced.

Facing uncertainties, both global and personal, we never know who will need us, do we?

When Others Need Us, How Do We Find Time for Our Own Needs?

While I was struggling to maintain my own fitness so I would be able to help care for an adult child, other women were struggling to find time for themselves while raising their families. From my own experience, I knew this is even more difficult if you're a parent who works outside the home.

Given demanding schedules, it's easy to focus on the immediate needs of our families—the next meal, the next load of laundry, getting the permission slip signed for school, running errands—and ignore our own needs. But no matter what we say to our children, our actions dictate the lessons they absorb and make their own. That's why the eating and exercise behavior of parents is critical to their children's long-term health.

Fighting Childhood Obesity

Childhood obesity is alarming and sad. Have you visited an elementary school lately? Have you seen how the overweight kids are isolated? Growing up is hard enough without the handicap of obesity. Everything I've read indicates that children who are overweight are likely to become overweight adults.

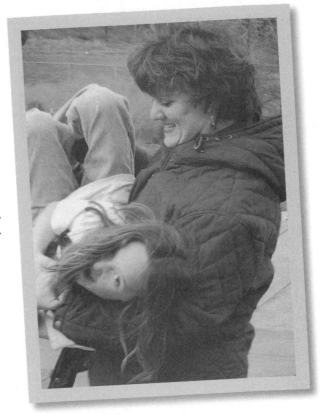

Laura Beavers is determined to set an example for children, starting with her own.

Setting an example is not only in the best interests of the parents but of their children as well. I didn't do a particularly good job myself, so perhaps that was why I was impressed with Laura Beavers.

Mom, You're So Skinny!

Others might search for a diet to make pounds magically disappear, but Laura tackled her goal using a tried-and-true formula—eating right and exercising. Moving to our area four years ago, Laura added pounds to an already overweight body when she found herself driving more and walking less. Weight on her 5'5" frame reached 250 pounds.

Watching a television show triggered a breakthrough for Laura. Dr. Phil, on Oprah Winfrey's show, suggested to an overweight guest that if she could find the cause of her unhappiness, the pounds might melt away. The dialogue made an impact on Laura. She realized that, unlike the unhappy guest, she was happy and had no barrier to getting fit. She began immediately.

To make changes in eating, Laura used the Mayo Clinic's free online service to keep a food diary and taught herself to eat only until she wasn't hungry. For exercise, she began lifting weights, spinning, dancing, walking, and playing basketball. The last time I checked on her, she'd lost sixty pounds and wanted to lose fifty more.

Despite working full time, parenting a seven-year-old, leading a scout group, and being a wife, Laura makes self-care a priority. In doing so, Laura becomes a role model for her daughter.

Laura's enthusiasm is contagious. "The greatest thrill about losing weight," she said, "is the increased energy I enjoy for everyday tasks— from tying my shoelaces to playing basketball with my daughter."

Laura's nicest compliment came when her daughter put her arms around her mom for a hug and said "Mom, you're so skinny!" With encouragement like that, Laura will reach her goal.

Setting a Better Example

I remember when I was Laura's age and my children were small like hers. I stood in front of the mirror in the bedroom, criticizing my body aloud and hating myself for being so fat.

"You're not fat, Mom," my younger son sweetly volunteered. "You're just short for your weight."

Bless his heart! He was doing his best to lift my spirits when in fact I should have been setting an example for him. I can't rewind the clock, but I can be an example for others today and going forward.

) (

Pride Goeth before a Fall

*We don't receive wisdom; we must discover it for ourselves
after a journey that no one can take for us or spare us.*
MARCEL PROUST

Barely a year had passed since I'd started my new lifestyle. I was eating healthfully, exercising, and controlling my weight. But I made the mistake of getting complacent. Little did I know that the fitness gods would test me to see if the new habits would dissolve under pressure.

I returned to Missouri to help my son-in-law cope with my daughter's recovery following her cardiac arrest two months earlier.

Becoming a Mom Again

For the next few weeks I was Jamie's caretaker as well as the homemaker for her husband and my three granddaughters. Maintaining my own regimen was a struggle. I needed to shower, get dressed, and finish my exercise program before anyone else was up; otherwise, events of the day overtook me.

The girls were awakened by their stepfather before he left for work at 7:00 AM. While they dressed and prepared for school, I coaxed Jamie out of bed and into the shower. The girls and I took turns reminding her to come out and get dressed. Without a sense of time or memory to guide her, Jamie might have stayed in the shower indefinitely.

During this hectic hour, the girls also watched their mother while I started a load of laundry. We left the house together. The girls went to school, and I drove Jamie to the rehabilitation center for therapy.

Keeping a Watchful Eye

Because Jamie had recovered physically, she was able to do anything, including driving a car. But with short-term memory still impaired, she would have been a hazard on the road. We had to watch her constantly, including keeping the car keys away from her.

Since Jamie looked like her former self, it was hard for her daughters to remember that she was no longer the same person. I reminded them that "Mom isn't herself right now." Sometimes we joked about our predicament. A little self-conscious about my levity, I told myself that laughter is better than crying.

The bitter Missouri cold, produced by snow and ice, made walking alone impossible. A thoughtful neighbor took me on two excursions—playing indoor tennis and hiking in the woods during a snowstorm. I was grateful for these carefree moments during such a nightmarish period.

Finding healthy eating was daunting. Everyone made fun of "Grandma's salad bar," which I set up nightly, hoping someone would join me. To avoid eating triple-cheese-with-sausage pizza, I bought cooked seafood, adding it to my nightly salad. There was predictability to my food, but at least I avoided fried chicken or worse.

Sugar Is My Downfall

I didn't always resist sweets and the snack foods the girls ate, although I knew adding pounds would increase my distress. Without a scale, I didn't know if I gained. At least my clothes were still fitting.

When I arrived home two weeks later, I slept seventeen of the first twenty-four hours. The next day I went to the gym and a yoga class. The following day I played tennis and was thrilled to be outdoors again. I was happy to cook "slow" food in my own kitchen once again.

The scale showed a four-pound gain—definitely a trend in the wrong direction!

Recovering My Self

I realized that my fitness habits were shaky. My daily food journal had to be expanded. Besides calories and exercise hours, I added a "well-being" category. I wrote down any actions I took to nurture myself, miracles I noticed, and areas that needed attention. For spiritual comfort, I returned to church. My husband and I invited easygoing friends over for lunch. Perspective gradually returned; perhaps self-discipline would follow.

Regaining Perspective

When we're struggling in our own lives, sometimes it is useful to see how others cope with even greater adversity. Inevitably that puts our own problems in perspective.

Sometimes after joining friends at our tennis clinic, I packed my gear away in my car and then noticed a young man loading his car. First he put in his tennis gear; then he loaded his wheelchair. Since he and I shared a love of tennis, I stopped to chat with him.

I was surprised to learn that Sean Conroy, at twenty-one, had taken up tennis only a few months earlier. That didn't stop him, though, from competing with opponents from the Nevada County Wheelchair Sports Association at Veterans Memorial Park in Grass Valley.

He told me he works out in two gyms—lifting weights and working on machines to keep his shoulders powerful. Because his shoulders do so much work in the wheelchair, they ache if he doesn't keep them strong.

He also shared his love of music. Sean plays the trumpet and performs on keyboard with a rock band. As if that doesn't keep him busy enough, he is also a full-time college student.

To keep his discipline, Sean makes exercise dates with friends. He wouldn't stand up a good friend and so even if he doesn't feel like working out, he keeps his word.

"Besides," he adds, "I don't feel as well when I don't exercise. I slow down and eat more. My energy declines and my body starts to hurt."

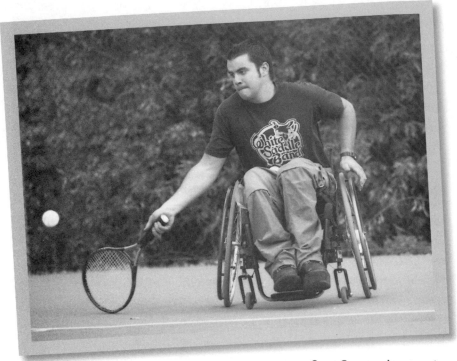

Sean Conroy plays tennis
with the intensity of a true athlete.

Sean has had plenty of time to develop self-discipline. Born with a tumor on his spinal cord, he's endured multiple surgeries on his back—six in the past year alone.

"Everybody has something to deal with," he says simply. Sean is definitely on top of his game—getting the most out of life!

So what, I asked myself, is your excuse? Are you willing to get the most out of your life for the time you have remaining? *Yes* was the spontaneous response.

) (

When the Apple Is Ripe

First it is necessary to stand on your own two feet.
But the minute a man finds himself in that position,
the next thing he should do is reach out his arms.

KRISTIN HUNTER

I decided to teach a class on fitness through the Wellness Center of the local hospital. I titled the class "Experiment in Living." Could I pass on to others what I'd learned? And what would I teach? The material would have to come from our combined needs. Talk about faith! Still, it was worth the gamble.

I decided to focus on one thing I'd learned: the key to fitness is managing one's internal thought processes. Practical and theoretical information would be useful, but unless the students changed their thinking, they would be trapped in a jail of their own making.

I would never have guessed that the star pupil would turn out to be Margaret Jonsen.

Arriving late at the first session, her gray hair flying, she interrupted the class to announce that the only reason she came was because her daughter had paid for the workshop. For her part, Margie was at the end of her rope. She had tried everything to get fit. As she bluntly stated, she had low expectations of the class—and of me, the instructor. Not stopping there, she tried to throw cold water on the enthusiasm of her classmates. If her words weren't enough, her dowdy clothes and disheveled hair told me a lot about how discouraged she felt.

The Big Experiment Did Not Fail After All

I looked around the classroom as she was making her aggressive remarks, wondering why I had agreed to lead it. How likely was it that twelve hours of instruction could alter decades of habits? Good thing, I reassured myself, the workshop is an "experiment." I couldn't guarantee results.

Collectively, among seven of us, we carried at least four hundred extra pounds. Being significantly overweight shortens women's lives by seven years and men's by six. If each person became fit, seventy years of added living were available, not to mention improving the quality of our remaining years and saving thousands of dollars in medical expenses.

My underlying theory was that "where the mind goes, the body follows." So each week we focused on thought processes. As the students practiced picking a perspective on fitness that best served their interests, better choices about food and exercise started to occur.

At the end of six weeks, and with reassurance that each person had a support system, I said good-bye. I was the reluctant parent seeing all her children leave home at once.

Reunion and Reckoning

We had our first reunion several weeks later. Of the original participants, one was continuing to take what she called baby steps, making small, incremental changes. The remaining six were making significant changes, which, if continued, would ultimately lead to fitness. As a group they had more than quadrupled their weekly exercise time from ten hours a week to more than forty. As a by-product of eating differently and exercising more, they had lost sixty-five pounds. They reported eating more fruits and vegetables and less sugar, caffeine, soft drinks, and processed foods.

One reported needing less sleep, another had organized and reduced her personal possessions, and another had been able to cut back on medications. To each other and to me, they looked more alive, healthy, and energetic.

Amazingly enough, the most recalcitrant student, Margaret Jonsen, was now the most enthusiastic. Her hair was cut in a sassy style. Even though she had many more pounds to lose, her clothes were more stylish, and she was now smiling. She had begun walking regularly with her daughter and was excited about her new cooking ideas. Her enthusiasm for new ways of eating and the energy she was getting from walking were contagious.

One by One

Do you remember the parable about the boy walking on the beach and tossing stranded starfish back into the ocean, one after the other? A cynical observer asked him why he bothered since there were hundreds to save. What difference would these puny efforts make in the course of the universe?

"Well," the boy replied, tossing yet another starfish, "it made a difference to that one."

My efforts too were puny. They wouldn't change the course of the "unfitness" epidemic. Surely, though, they mattered to these seven people whose lives had been altered by our experiment.

At this point I was both the teacher and the student on the fitness journey. Sometimes I was the one who taught; other times I was the one who needed to be shown the way. One of my guides, even though he was legally blind, gave me a remarkable vision of what was possible.

Seeing the Value in Staying Fit

I met David Ayala by accident, literally. I lost my footing working with weights in the gym and nearly bumped into a tall man working out next to me. Unlike me, he was particularly well balanced. Watching him, I realized that he had limited vision. Curious about how he kept himself so fit, I introduced myself and started asking questions. Although he considered his regimen ordinary, it was anything but. I had to wonder, If someone with David's physical challenges could accomplish so much, what were we couch potatoes waiting for?

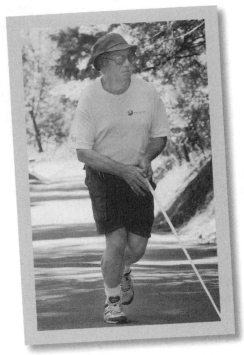

David Ayala takes his daily four-mile walk along a local trail.

Blinded by an inherited condition, David Ayala, at fifty-eight, reports a lifelong commitment to staying fit. He isn't disciplined so much as practical: "I feel better when I'm in shape," he explains.

David ran track in high school in the early sixties and just kept on running. "Some friends," he says, "got into their cars at sixteen, never left, and now wonder why they have back problems."

David isn't happy unless he's moving. He likes to feel light on his feet from balance exercises, weights, the Stairmaster, jogging, and aerobic exercises. Otherwise, he says, "I feel grumpy."

Without vision, balance and fitness are essential yet more difficult to achieve. "If you doubt me," he says, "try balancing on one leg with [your] eyes closed. Now try balancing on one leg to see how important strength is." David focused on building up both.

He also manages his weight. He had started the year at 200 pounds, but in two months he'd lost a total of 10 and was now down to 190. He wanted to reach 185.

David's weekly regimen is two to three one-hour gym workouts, plus jogging. His white cane alerts him to objects in a path that takes him on a lightly traveled four-mile route.

If each of us could see staying fit through David's eyes, perhaps our own self-care vision would be clearer.

Everyone Around Me Becomes My Teacher

David, however, was only one of many people from our town who were inspiring me. Almost daily someone still stopped me as I bought groceries, pumped gas, or walked along a trail.

One woman, Sandee Buckmaster, went on daily walks until she had dropped 135 pounds. Cyd Sharkey decided to shape up for her forty-seventh birthday; she wanted to set a good example for her daughters. She began attending Weight Watchers meetings and exercising daily and moved quickly toward her fitness goals.

Jim Simmons reinvented himself at sixty-three. He trimmed down through changes in eating, gave up alcohol, and started climbing mountains. Tim Koumb, a nurse, was having trouble moving around. When his weight peaked at 304 pounds, he decided enough was enough. He bought exercise equipment, started working out, and changed his eating. At forty, he had brought his weight down to 215 pounds.

Richard DicKard, a dentist, practiced tai chi, or "moving meditation," as he called it, to keep in shape and prevent back problems. It also improved his balance, increased his flexibility, and strengthened his bones and muscles.

Betty Klein at sixty-eight was an undiagnosed diabetic until a routine test picked up her problem. Five years later she'd taken off forty-seven pounds by eating differently and exercising daily.

As I listened to their stories, I felt my own courage rise again. I realized that once we saw others making changes, all of us had more hope that we, too, could change. We benefited from knowing about one another's successes.

Was I in a beautiful orchard filled with ripening apples? Was now the time for others to commit to fitness just as I had?

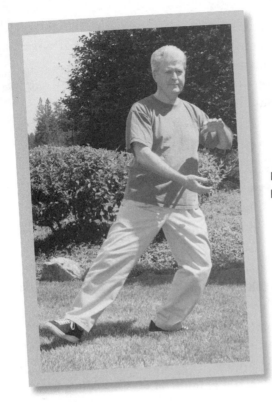

**Richard DicKard
practices tai chi.**

The idea of a group effort began percolating in my brain even as I tried to resist it. How could I possibly take on one more commitment? I could barely keep up with my current writing and exercise schedule! Plus I liked to cook and sew and spend time with my family.

I needed to make a trip back to Missouri to help with Jamie's care and give her husband and children a break. Jamie's memory remained impaired so that by noon she couldn't remember what she'd eaten for breakfast or, for that matter, if she'd eaten at all. I also needed to bring her children to California to give them a break from caretaking for their mom and a chance just to be kids again. And, of course, there were other offspring to see, an aging mother in Iowa to visit, friends to entertain, obligations at church, tennis clinics, and vacation trips with my husband.

Where was the retire in retirement?

At the same time, if the apples were ripe, should I pick them?

PART 3

From a Private to a Public Matter

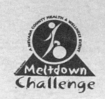

Ordinary People
Doing
Extraordinary
Things

Why not go out on a limb?
Isn't that where the fruit is?

FRANK SCULLY

) (

Since I'd requested the appointment, I could hardly cancel the meeting with Mike Carville, the general manager and owner of the South Yuba Fitness Club in Nevada City. I was coming down with a cold, and a sore throat and fatigue made me want to curl up in front of a fire on this gray November afternoon. Still, I dragged myself out of the house and drove the seven miles down Banner Mountain through the tall pine trees. Leaves on an occasional oak tree had started to turn orange and red from the first chilly nights of fall. At the club I wearily climbed the stairs to the second-floor office, where I found Mike working at his computer.

Despite threatening rain, we decided to walk while we talked. I had a vague idea about a community fitness project that I'd been wanting to pursue with Mike. (The notion had seemed clearer a few days earlier when I'd felt perkier.) Since Mike was the general manager of my fitness club, he seemed like the logical person to approach. Also, he was a Certified Personal Fitness Trainer, as designated by the National Academy of Sports Medicine, the global authority in fitness-related certification. Over the past five years more than twenty-three hundred people had attended "Getting Started," his ten-week conditioning and weight-loss program. From the programs his club offered, I knew that he, too, felt obesity was the number one national health issue.

With only the germ of an idea in my mind, I set out with him on as much of a hike as I could muster.

An hour later Mike and I had a tentative plan. His club would provide a meeting room and act as host for the group fitness project. The purpose would be to educate participants on the value of becoming fit. People would be encouraged to make healthy lifestyle choices and to have fun together while doing it. One idea built on another, until Mike and I had outlined what we'd already started calling the "Nevada County Meltdown." Our excitement built as ideas and plans unfolded between us. We could help change our community!

Driving home, I felt reenergized. The cold symptoms that had nearly kept me away from our meeting had completely disappeared.

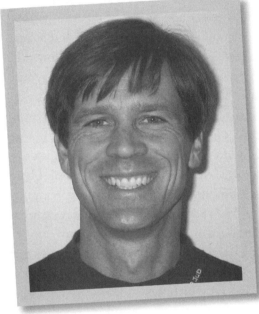

Mike Carville is blessed with energy and high spirits. He and I form an instant partnership— we're not certain what we are going to do, but whatever we do, we'll do it with enthusiasm.

) (

The Nevada County Meltdown Takes Shape

*You sort of start thinking anything's possible
if you've got enough nerve.*

J. K. ROWLING

Once Mike and I had a name for the project and a tentative plan, the pieces started falling into place. We'd meet weekly, attendance would be optional, and people could continue to join throughout the program. Mike made a generous offer: to promote fitness during the eight-week program, participants would be allowed free use of his fitness center.

We'd heard of a similar "meltdown" fitness project in Garden City, Kansas. Although neither of us knew much about their program, which we'd seen in a brief newspaper article, we were untroubled by our lack of knowledge. We would create a unique program as we went along. Any critics could be silenced by explaining that this was a work in progress.

We also agreed that the program would be free and noncommercial. Moreover, no specific diet or exercise regimen would be prescribed; rather, we would encourage people to find their personal and unique eating and exercise regimen, hopefully one they would maintain for a lifetime.

Both of us believed strongly that a support system helps people make changes. Consequently, we would organize participants into teams of five; however, we'd be flexible. Teams could have as many members as they wanted, as long as they were organized and had a system for communication. Friendly rivalry between teams, churches, even towns (Grass Valley and Nevada City have had a friendly rivalry for 150 years) would be encouraged.

Thanksgiving was fast approaching, and the winter holidays wouldn't be far behind. That meant family visits and houseguests for me and extra club activities for Mike. We already had full calendars, so we adopted our first policy: "No deadly planning meetings!" All work would be done by phone and e-mail.

Mike and I decided we would lead the Meltdown until we could find a person or service group to take over. While the search for our replacement was going on, we could be lining up carefully selected professionals with specialized expertise on topics of interest—exercise, medical issues, and nutrition—for the weekly presentations. My role would be to cover practical aspects based on my recent weight-loss experience.

Sessions would be held in the evening, during after-work hours. At the first session we'd arrange carpooling for people who didn't drive at night. Sessions would begin promptly at 7:00 PM, be focused and energetic, and end before 9:00.

The first event would be spent on organization and getting started. At subsequent sessions we'd spend the first hour using a town hall format to report individual and team results and then follow with a short informational presentation. Then we'd respond to questions, provide answers, and end promptly.

We had two quick decisions to make—when to start and when to end. We picked a starting date of the first Tuesday of the new year, January 6, and an ending date of the last Tuesday in February. This would give us time to announce the program, and eight weeks would be long enough, we hoped, for participants to adopt new lifestyle behaviors.

I would make my presentation at the beginning of the series and would attend the meetings for the first four weeks. After that I was scheduled for a vacation with my husband in Kauai. By that time, Mike's wife would be close to her due date for their baby, but he still wanted to proceed even though he knew he might end up carrying the whole load in the final four meetings.

Open to the Public and Free

To find out if people were interested, I volunteered to write an article for the *Union* issuing a public invitation. I'd also ask for an individual or service group to head the project and for people to contribute specialized expertise.

Mike would distribute information about the fledgling program to his club's members. Anticipating the new year, he had already planned a December radio promotion for his club; that campaign would be steered to promote the Meltdown.

With a general plan, a handshake, and nothing in writing, Mike and I went to work.

If Not Us, Who? If Not Now, When?

The article inviting readers to join in a community fitness effort appeared in early November. I began with a simple question: "If not us, who? If not now, when?"

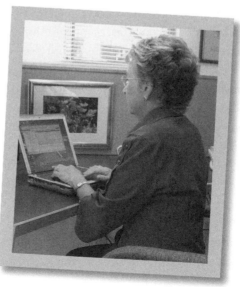

I was uncertain if anyone would respond to the invitation. Or if they did, where would I find volunteers to help?

I shared information about offers local experts were already making to the project. The hospital dietitian wanted to make a presentation on nutrition. A fitness club was donating passes to participants and providing a meeting room. A physical therapist would teach us safe exercise regimens. A hairstylist would provide makeovers to the winning team.

Then I asked who was interested in participating. Could they get five people together? From church? From work? Friends and family members? Then I added my e-mail address, wondering if I would hear from anyone.

The day the article appeared, my inbox registered sixteen inquiries. People wanted to join; specialists wanted to lend their expertise. But no one stepped forward to head the project. Mike and I realized that for better or worse, we would have to make it happen. The word was out, and now we couldn't back out of the project even if we wanted to. The clock had already begun ticking.

Six Weeks to Go

A community group focusing on health and wellness invited us to their December meeting. This coalition included health care educators; a city recreation department employee; the public relations manager from the local hospital; a fitness center owner; a physician; representatives from the alternative health care community, the hospital's Wellness Center, and the United Way; and the county superintendent of schools.

This coalition had set out to develop and support organized community health actions. They were enthusiastic about our Meltdown idea and immediately went to work. Endorsements from United Way, the *Union*, and Sierra Nevada Memorial Hospital enhanced the Meltdown's credibility. One coalition member, Ruth Bedwell, said she would work to get January and February proclaimed as official Meltdown months by the city councils of Grass Valley and Nevada City and by the Nevada County Board of Supervisors.

The community assessment project director, Lori Burkart Frank, volunteered to distribute our flyers at Weight Watchers meetings. Gary Cooke, the public relations manager for the hospital, provided us with a list of contacts so we could alert the media. He also promised to devote the hospital's December radio commercials to promoting the Meltdown.

With this much support, I had little problem persuading speakers to donate their time and expertise. Instructions went out to each: inform and inspire us in twenty minutes or less!

Five Weeks to Go

Community approval notwithstanding, the real test would be participation. Would residents support such an event? Would they come out on stormy weeknights in the middle of a rainy winter to address fitness issues?

In mid-December, I wrote a second article for the *Union* inviting participation in the Meltdown. The dozens of e-mails I received in response showed me we would need a lot more free gym passes. I had a new urgent task—to persuade all fitness centers in the county to participate.

Four Weeks to Go

As word of the coming event spread, six more facilities (Fast and Fit, Courthouse Athletic Club, Curves of Nevada City and Grass Valley, Curves of Penn Valley, Jazzercise, and Club Sierra) agreed to give free passes to Meltdown participants. The entire county was covered! I sent out a letter that began and ended with the same plea: "Please bring an ample supply of guest passes. We don't want to disappoint the participants who show up. It will be better for us to have too many passes than too few."

Three Weeks to Go

Momentum was building. Suzie Daggett, a well-known spokesperson in the local alternative health community, invited me to appear on her show on the community television channel. Another health coalition member, Debbie Wagner, coordinator of the Sierra Nevada Memorial Hospital's Wellness Center, sent out an e-mail to several hundred physicians.

With this growing publicity, inquiries were pouring in. My e-mail inbox was now flooded. How could I possibly answer everybody's questions? Then Lori Burkart Frank of United Way stepped in, developing a question-and-answer sheet to hand out.

One inquiry came from Dena Nick, a mother of six, who called to talk about the heavy demands of parenting. She worried that she would take valuable time away from her family if she attended an evening meeting every week. I tried to persuade her that taking care of herself was the foundation of being a good parent. Instead of feeling guilty about caring for her own fitness, she would be setting the example that her children needed.

Two Weeks to Go

Three local radio stations, KNCO, KNCO-Star, and KVMR, began broadcasting public service announcements and brought me in for on-air interviews to promote the Meltdown. The Grass Valley and Nevada City chambers of commerce also mentioned the Meltdown in weekly radio broadcasts. Dixie Redfearn at the *Union* added teasers about the Meltdown to her daily column to pique public interest.

The staff at the South Yuba Club designed a colorful logo and flyer to be inserted in the *Union* alerting subscribers to the event. I wasn't sure there'd be any interest, but I sent a press release to Sacramento-area newspapers and television stations. Then I watched with amazement as each individual and group promoted the Meltdown in their own venues. The word was spreading on a network of friendships and associations, and buzz in town was building with little central direction.

Was the Meltdown an idea whose time had come?

My third article on the Meltdown appeared on New Year's Day in the *Union* and triggered an avalanche of inquiries. I was both excited and apprehensive. Many people were expressing interest, but would they actually attend a meeting? How could we estimate attendance? How many people did a single e-mail represent? One person? A team of five? We knew that teams were organizing, but how many people were on a team? What impact would a projected winter storm have? I was too anxious to sleep. What had I done?

One Week to Go

The original idea was to hold the meeting at the South Yuba Club exercise studio, which accommodates fifty people. Back in November this had seemed more than adequate. Even so, I kept asking myself, "What if?"—particularly as e-mails kept pouring in.

Mike tried to calm my anxiety. He wasn't convinced we needed more room, but he did agree to relocate to the Nevada Union High School, with seating for 450. Now I worried that only a dozen people would show up and I'd look like a woman suffering from serious delusions of grandeur. Nonetheless, I started lining up volunteers to help in case we had a larger-than-expected turnout.

What Would We Do in the First Meeting?

With one week to go, we needed a little more structure. The idea of the Meltdown was to promote fitness, but how would we know if we were achieving our goal? People might come for many reasons—to gain flexibility, improve balance, increase stamina, or improve a medical condition, or just for the free eight-week pass to their neighborhood fitness center. We couldn't measure fitness in each of these categories. For simplicity, then, we chose to measure weight loss.

We'd need to obtain starting and ending weights for teams. This information could be updated at future meetings and used as the basis for awarding prizes at the end. We designed a team registration form to record the weights of team members and then set up an e-mail system for communicating updates. A Web mistress at the *Union*, Dayna Amboy, started creating a Web site.

We would have a lot to accomplish on the first night. Besides introducing the Meltdown, we needed to get everyone assigned to a team, designate each team's captain, review the ground rules, collect current team weights, set team goals, distribute free passes from the clubs and fitness centers, give out information on how to start a fitness program, set up an e-mail communication system, and announce plans for the next meeting. Whew!

I'd had some experience organizing large groups of people in one of my consulting jobs, and I remembered that seating people in groups helped them get to work faster. So we divided the county into four geographical parts and organized seating in the auditorium so volunteer ushers could direct participants to their area. Besides helping people form teams, sitting close to neighbors would help them find carpools for subsequent meetings.

I also knew from working with training seminars for large groups that participants often needed help to get organized. To accomplish that task, I designated one set of volunteers as team creators. Their job would be to circulate around the room and make sure everyone found a team. Once a team was formed, a second set of volunteer facilitators would help teams choose a captain and establish individual and team goals.

Gyms and fitness center owners would set up tables in the lobby with a supply of passes, sign-up sheets, and releases. Mike would be our first night's speaker, outlining the sobering implications of the obesity/fitness problem and offering guidelines for safe exercise.

To make the evening go as smoothly as possible, using my background in personnel work, I quickly wrote job descriptions for the team creators and facilitators. I also appointed a volunteer coordinator and put him fully in charge. I set up an e-mail system for collecting and reporting team weight information using the model I was familiar with from several years of operating retail stores.

Would two, twenty, or two hundred people show up? None of us had any idea. Rushing with last-minute details, anxious about how large it might be—or how small—we did our best to be prepared.

Twenty-four Hours to Go

We were taking a huge leap of faith. Suspended between terror and exhilaration, I waited for the first event.

Riding the Tiger

Somebody has to do something,
and it's just incredibly pathetic that it has to be us.

JERRY GARCIA

My husband, who had minimal interest in getting fit and losing weight, decided to come to the first meeting to support me. As we drove the fifteen minutes to our local high school theater, I felt like a lamb being led to slaughter.

As the catalyst for the Meltdown, I would make the opening remarks. For the first time, I would publicly articulate the collective vision that was spontaneously emerging in our community. Together we could become "the fittest little county in the nation." Just as my weight-loss story had been a catalyst for others, our community could become a catalyst for the nation. Would anybody come to listen and confirm the vision?

Earlier in the day, I had attended a meeting of the county board of supervisors to accept their proclamation of January and February 2004 as official Nevada County Meltdown months. In our county, supervisors typically line up on opposite sides of any issue. But the Meltdown proclamation was something board members could agree on. They unanimously offered their support, and each supervisor took a turn emphasizing the importance of committing to fitness. Some were concerned about the impact of obesity on individuals; others talked of the financial implications if obesity wasn't addressed.

The proclamation was wonderful, but the real test was about to take place. Would anyone show up for the meeting?

Let the Fun Begin

Setup for the meeting was scheduled to begin at 6:00 PM, with doors opening to the public at 6:30. When I arrived at 5:30, to my astonishment, the parking lot was already nearly full. True to their word, the gyms and fitness centers were setting up tables in the lobby; Mike was checking out the video equipment. Volunteers were busy going over their assignments, and signs had been posted to direct participants to their seats.

The only surprise was the steady stream of guests, who were filling seats so rapidly that ushers could barely steer people to the right geographic sections. By 6:30 the theater, which seats 450, was full. By 6:45 participants were sitting on the stage floor. Steps in the aisles were filling up as people sat down wherever they could. People were starting to stand three and four deep in the back of the theater. The lobby was jammed full; still more people were trying to get in.

Concerned about safety, ushers started turning residents away around 6:50 PM. Later we learned that traffic was backed up a mile or more on either side of the high school. Our best estimate is that between seven and eight hundred people jammed into the theater that night, and several hundred more were turned away.

Mike Carville and I proudly pose for a photograph after accepting the proclamation from the Nevada County Board of Supervisors.

We are jammed together. Some sit in aisles; others stand at the back as I begin the program.

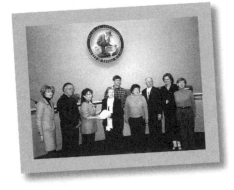
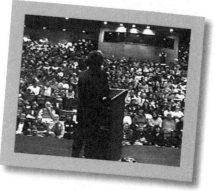

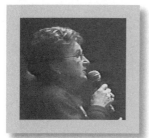

Once I begin talking, I start tingling with excitement. In that instant, I knew what we would accomplish together—I could feel it in the room.

The atmosphere in the theater was one of high spirits. Seeing neighbors and friends in the same condition—wanting to get fit, needing to lose a few pounds—brought smiles and laughter all around. If we had gotten ourselves into this state, we could have a good time getting out of it. We could have fun while we were getting fit! Adding to the excitement was the unexpected appearance of a KCRA Sacramento television news team.

Stretched to the maximum but thrilled at the response, Mike and I worked our way through the program. My opening remarks were taped for broadcast on the ten o'clock Sacramento news. Then Mike took the stage.

"Getting Started on Your Fitness Journey"

Mike told participants that the "space between our ears" was the hardest part of the body to condition. That's why, he said, the first step was to make a conscious decision to get fit. He encouraged participants to eat affirmatively—to develop a nutrition plan that responds to each person's unique body.

Regarding exercise, Mike said both strength and cardiovascular conditioning are important. While cardiovascular exercise burns calories, strength training is needed to increase metabolism. He encouraged us

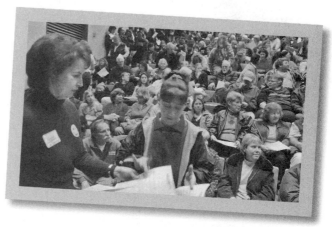

Gayle Lossman, personal trainer, helps a participant find teammates.

to approach our project positively and realistically. Instead of trying to cross the river in a single leap, we might use steppingstones, minigoals, so we could celebrate our successes. "Progress," he said, "not perfection, is the goal."

Getting Organized and Creating Teams

Then we went over the ground rules for the remaining eight weeks, including how to be eligible for team prizes at the end. We weren't going to require regular attendance at meetings to be eligible for prizes, but, to be fair, we did require that teams compete from the first session. Each person would report his or her starting weight, and then we would calculate pounds lost right before the last meeting. We would tabulate weight-loss results on a per-person basis so that a team of three could be compared to a team of one or a team of five. With most of the mechanics taken care of, we began organizing teams.

Such excitement! The room filled with the sound of hundreds of voices as names and e-mail addresses were exchanged, weights totaled, and captains identified. Some teams had come intact—a group from work or church or a group of neighbors. Others had come to the meeting alone or with a friend. Working quickly, we matched up individuals with neighbors. Once teams were formed, volunteer facilitators helped

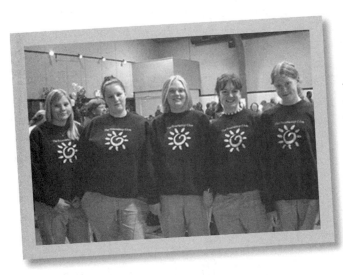

Teenage girls from the Friendship Club formed their own team. Pictured from left to right are Trista, Corina, Jodi, Alisha, and Hannah.

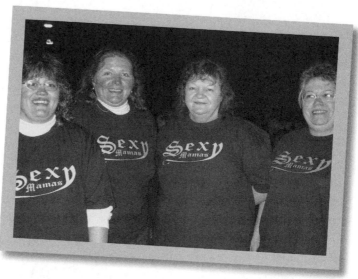

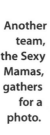

Another team, the Sexy Mamas, gathers for a photo.

members pick a system of communication and then a captain. We were a community in action!

All our preparation had paid off. Thanks to dozens of volunteers, by the end of the evening an amazing 136 teams totaling 651 people had been registered. Hundreds of passes to gyms and fitness centers had been distributed so that participants could begin exercise the following day.

A feedback loop was in place. Participants agreed to weigh themselves every Sunday night and forward their weight losses to their team captains. Team captains would then e-mail their team's weekly weight loss to Mike or me on Monday. We would total the amount and report results at our Tuesday session. We would also post results on our Web site and report them each week in the Friday issue of the *Union*.

With 651 people to keep track of, I quickly realized that a staggering amount of work was needed to record team results. Someone would need to spend hours each week at a computer, collecting e-mails and tabulating results on spreadsheets. Just then Dale Boothby, a pharmacist with exceptional computer skills, stepped forward to tackle this volunteer project. I heaved a sigh of relief no doubt heard in the next county. Surely this project was blessed!

Finding a Meeting Place

But one obvious problem remained. At the opening night we couldn't announce future meeting locations because we didn't know where they would be held. Where would we find a hall bigger than the high school auditorium? Did we even need such a place, or would attendance fall off now that the free passes had been handed out? Nor could we announce the location for a makeup session on Saturday for those who had been turned away from Tuesday's meeting. Would anyone come out on a busy weekend morning? The best we could do was to tell participants to check the newspaper and local radio stations for announcements on the new location and hope the word got out.

Once home, I kicked off my shoes and sank into a chair. What an evening! After my husband and I watched the report on the Meltdown on the nightly news, I was hyped. Despite the late hour, I called my son Marc in San Francisco. Eager to share the evening's excitement, I also wanted to get his advice about how to proceed. He'd been through law school, and I needed the assistance of his clear thinking and his humor.

And then began another benefit of the Nevada County Meltdown. From that point on I consulted with my son daily, sometimes several times a day; the child was coaching the parent. He always stayed one step ahead of me and so helped me anticipate what was needed next. Developing a professional relationship with my son was an unexpected by-product of the Meltdown, one that continues today.

In bed that night and unable to sleep, I stared wide-eyed at the ceiling. What in the world had happened? Were there really that many people wanting to get fit? Where would we meet next week? If I had been anxious before, now I was in a state of utter panic.

My husband's last words before sleep were hardly reassuring. "Remember," he said, "once you ride the tiger, you can't get off."

Achieving Our Personal Best

Real glory springs from the silent conquest of ourselves.

JOSEPH P. THOMPSON

The next day, Wednesday, Mike and I started scrambling. We forced ourselves to remain calm in the middle of the panic to find a new venue—quickly! Plus, we didn't have any formal organization or insurance. Even if we found a place, could we get the word out in time?

A member of the health coalition, Sharyn Turner, a school nurse in the office of the county superintendent of schools, called me to suggest that we use the high school cafeteria from then on; the room could hold 950 people. Surely, she said, that would be enough space. Mike and I agreed, figuring that much of the first night's excitement had been triggered by the free passes, and attendance would probably fall off.

Sharyn quickly obtained the necessary approvals and support of the high school staff, including the custodial workers who would supervise the volunteers as they arranged seating and tables for the meeting. She solved a very big problem with a few well-placed phone calls.

Through e-mail, radio, and newspaper announcements, we spread the word that Saturday's event and future sessions would be held at the Nevada Union High School's cafeteria. On Saturday we would also be able to distribute more free passes, thanks to the generosity of the fitness clubs. We didn't think many people would come, though, since Saturdays are sacrosanct for working people, time to run errands and do chores.

Wrong Again!

Once again we were stunned when several hundred people showed up. Volunteers had arranged seating for two hundred, and twenty minutes before the program started every seat was full. Dozens more teams were registered, and again we handed out several hundred free passes to fitness centers.

By Sunday morning I wanted to rest from the work of producing and coordinating two events in the prior week. Instead, I tackled the second week's program, only three days away. Realizing the mountain of work to be done each week, Mike and I designated point persons in key areas—volunteer coordination, event production, media relations, statistics, and programs.

Word trickled back to us that the buzz about the Meltdown was heard everywhere in town. Pastors were even mentioning it in church services. Participants were e-mailing their relatives in different parts of the country.

Our local radio stations featured Meltdown team members on their talk shows, and I began giving weekly radio reports on Monday mornings. The *Union*'s Web site for the Meltdown was already up and running, so participants could find exercise partners, boast about team results, share low-cal recipes, check on each other's progress, learn about the new prizes, and get information about coming events.

I was given a full newspaper page to fill each Friday with Meltdown topics—our progress in terms of pounds lost, stories and photographs of participants, my personal column, inspirational quotes, and articles on fitness written by local experts. In addition, I continued my weekly column sharing the story of my own quest for fitness.

My husband's prediction was correct—I couldn't get off the tiger!

Mike and I had mixed feelings about this ever-expanding undertaking. Fewer people would have made the project more manageable, a definite plus for each of us. At the same time, we felt an obligation to include as many people as possible. We'd just have to see what the next session brought.

Our Efforts Start to Get Noticed

Even though the second event wouldn't start until 7:00 PM, I needed to be dressed and ready by midafternoon. A television reporter from KOVR television in Sacramento wanted to interview me at home. They'd also be covering the event that evening for a segment on the late evening news.

I had no time to get nervous about the interview. I was too busy being nervous about giving that evening's talk—with PowerPoint presentation technology, which I'd never used before. The taping session with the reporter turned out to be relaxed and fun. I didn't mind that the picture of me they used to start the story was my "before" picture. That wasn't "me" anymore. If it helped others to see the changes I had made, I was willing to let it be broadcast to thousands. The interview was over in time for me to grab a banana as I raced out the door for our second Meltdown weekly meeting.

Arriving at the high school cafeteria at 5:00 PM, I was both reassured and touched by the presence of the high school janitors, who were working overtime to set up the room. Volunteers were setting up the sound equipment and testing the PowerPoint system.

Benches in the cavernous room quickly filled with early arrivals. Other participants walked laps around the room to log exercise minutes. A couple of nurses set up free blood pressure and body fat testing, and a line quickly formed at their table. By 6:30 the 950 seats were completely filled, with late arrivals again forced to stand four and five rows deep around the room.

Again spirits were high. We celebrated our successes. In one week we had added thirty more teams, and the Meltdown now totaled 791 participants. People also had started losing weight—1,687 pounds reported lost so far. The crowd greeted each announcement with raucous laughter, whistles, yelling, and cheers. If enthusiasm was what it took to lose weight, we were well on our way to success!

I knew from my own weight-loss months that people are motivated by hearing the stories of others, so we gave time for people to tell their experiences. When Kerry Arnett, the mayor of Nevada City, stood up in front of the microphone and unequivocally committed himself to losing weight, the audience cheered wildly.

Then it was my turn to speak.

Realizing Our Personal Best

How could I condense forty years of professional and real-life experience into fifteen minutes? I wanted to tell them everything I'd learned in my years as a stay-at-home mom, a high school teacher, a senior administrator at the University of California, a business consultant, and a chief executive officer of several companies. Every skill I'd ever honed was needed now, in this new job I'd inadvertently created—catalyst for the Meltdown.

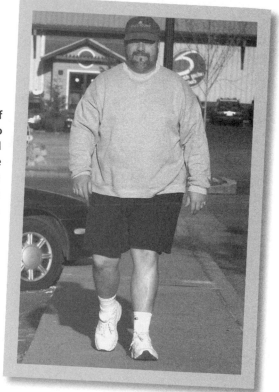

Kerry Arnett, mayor of Nevada City, pledged to tackle his personal and overdue project to lose weight and become more fit. He heads out on his daily walk.

I began with my own story—and the moment of truth when I stepped on the scale and it broke. Looking at the faces in the room, I asked each person to make a conscious decision about their own personal future: to take personal and immediate responsibility for the care and nurturing of their bodies.

"Each of us," I stated, "must consciously choose what to change in our life and how we will change it. In some cases, that will mean adding elements that are not present; in other cases, it will mean removing or substituting."

"Redefine your self-image," I encouraged the crowd. "Start saying to yourself, 'I'm the kind of person who . . .' and fill in the blank with something positive." I gave an example: "Instead of 'I'm the kind of person who loves a big evening meal,' say, 'I'm the kind of person who likes to eat healthfully.' By using constructive language to describe ourselves, we can enhance our image." This was, I added, important because so many of us were hard on ourselves for having gotten so overweight and out of shape.

I also tried to dispel the old notion that taking care of ourselves is selfish. "It's not narcissistic to tend your own health and physical well-being," I asserted. "It's not 'me first' to take care of your body. It's 'me too.'"

I also delivered the bad news—that there was no "there" there in our fitness journey. There was no destination and no point of arrival. We were on a lifetime quest. I encouraged them to make their travels exhilarating and to enjoy each moment. Peaks and valleys, successes and setbacks, I assured them, were part of the trip. When the going got tough, I advised, "Don't quit! Instead, recommit."

The Professional Human Being

I concluded with a notion I had taken from Epictetus, the Greek philosopher who suggested we live as "professional human beings." "When you are deciding what to eat, what to drink, or whether to exercise," I advised, "ask yourself what is in your best interest. Don't ask what you want—you know what you want! Ask instead what decision will serve you best." I was confident that if participants could see their best interests clearly, they would consistently and easily make choices that supported their fitness goals.

"Laugh a lot!" I ended. When I finished, I saw sparkling eyes and heard enthusiastic applause. Maybe what I'd gleaned in forty years of both professional work and work on myself could indeed be useful to others.

My presence, however, was a far more powerful testimonial than my ideas. Because I had made dramatic changes and become happier and healthier, I opened up possibilities for each one of them. I offered hope that they could realize their dreams as well. That awareness triggered a joyful sense of excitement—I wanted to hug each one of them.

Media Hounds Sign Up

Before the end of the evening, more than one hundred volunteers signed up to talk to the media and share their stories. We also scheduled our first midweek community walk to take place at the local high school. Dozens of people wanted more chances not only to exercise but also to meet their neighbors and make new friends. More teams were registered and free fitness center passes handed out. Finally the evening ended.

But I couldn't go home yet. Eric Bailey, a reporter from the *Los Angeles Times*, came forward to grill me. He was amazed at the size of the turnout—well over a thousand people!—and shared his own desire to drop a few pounds. He had come to write an article and left inspired to make changes in his own life. Our program was making an impact even on people hundreds of miles away!

A Flock Without a Pasture

Everyone had said that participation would fall off after the first week, and I had believed them, knowing the history of failure with projects involving weight loss. But instead of declining, participation was increasing. The implications were frighteningly wonderful. We needed yet a larger venue both to seat people and also to have more space for pre-event activities. But where? I felt like a shepherd with a flock too large for the pasture.

When my husband and I got to our car after the second week's event, we found a flyer on the windshield promoting a quick fix for weight loss. Flyers had been placed on all the cars as far as the eye could see. We'd promised a noncommercial program, and now someone was trying to exploit our event. I made a mental note to apologize to the crowd at our next session.

The Law of Unintended Consequences

The following day I received three memorable phone calls. The first was from a participant who was searching for a bath scale so she could report her weight to her captain. She had searched in local hardware stores, discount stores, and drug stores, she said, and not a scale was to be found. She wanted me to know that she was going to drive to Roseville, an hour away, and bring back a quantity to sell to her friends. I laughed when I hung up the phone.

The second phone call was from Bill Dempsey, the supervising volunteer at the community's Interfaith Food Ministry. "What," he asked, "do you want us to do with all this bread and pastry?"

I asked why he was calling me.

"Well," he said, "normally the two-day-old bread and pastry from the grocery stores is quickly distributed to our clients. But since the Meltdown started, the stores are not selling much bread and pastry. They're bringing truckloads of the stuff to our center. What we are supposed to do with it?" Once again I hung up the phone laughing.

Then I had to get more serious. Another event needed to be planned, a new venue located. Media requests both local and statewide were accumulating. Each reporter needed background information as well as people to interview. Plus I needed to keep my own fitness program going. Where to begin?

In that moment the phone rang for the third time.

"Hello," the woman said. "My name is Emi Sakai. I'm your neighbor a mile or so away, and I thought you might need some help."

"How soon can you come over?" I asked, trying to keep the desperation out of my voice.

"How about now?" she replied.

Within the hour Emi arrived, bringing years of experience as an executive assistant. By the end of our first session together, she had organized my home office. Equally important, she was a calming presence and a wonderful companion. Instantly she was indispensable. I began sharing each day's developments with her.

Although she operated in the background, Emi became essential to the success of the Meltdown. She fielded dozens of e-mails and kept track of each detail. She also showed up at meetings armed with supplies—all the flyers, name tags, and paraphernalia it took to orchestrate an event for a thousand people.

Once again I was in awe of the forces at work that bring forth such remarkable people at the exact moment when they are needed. Becoming aware of helpful forces did not prevent me from worrying, but it did give me humility about my own contribution.

Would others continue to step forward when needed?

The Circle Keeps Expanding

Be bold, and mighty powers will come to your aid.

BASIL KING

The following day Jon Katis, one of the fitness club managers, called and suggested the Nevada County Fairgrounds main hall for future meetings. The exhibit hall was well known and centrally located. It had what we needed—ample parking, clean restrooms, and a huge interior space that could accommodate our growing crowd.

Jon was a member of the local Rotary Club, which had agreed to provide us free liability insurance to use the hall. With the cooperation of Ed Scofield, fairgrounds manager, we gained permission to use the facility. I jumped at the opportunity to schedule subsequent meetings at a single location. One huge problem solved!

Jon reminded me of the downside. The fairgrounds had only four hundred chairs available for our use. We needed over nine hundred.

"How can we get more chairs?" I asked.

"I'll get some guys to truck in a few hundred chairs from the Grass Valley Methodist Church," he volunteered.

"Truck them in?" I asked incredulously.

"Yes, I'm sure we can find someone to take this one on. I'd also like to help out with the PA system in the fairgrounds hall," he added. "It can be a little tricky sometimes."

At that moment Jon had become our point person for facility management, although it was a week or so before I had the courage to tell him about his permanent assignment.

Establishing Our Management Structure

The next phone call was to Fred Lossman, coordinator of volunteers. Fred would have to recruit people for this backbreaking chair assignment. He graciously took on the task but insisted—I could nearly see his tongue planted firmly in cheek—that from this point forward his title would have to be Chair Man of the Board.

Working with all the point people, Mike and I continued our policy of "no meetings." Everything had to be done by e-mail or phone. Decisions were made on the spot by the point person. Mike and I squeezed in quick phone calls as needed and managed to meet an hour before each event to review the details of the program.

Now a second volunteer started working in my home office, to take care of statistics and e-mail, which continued to pour in. About 95 percent of the statistics were being reported on time, which meant that, with more help, we could keep our Web site current.

An Angel Appears at Round Table Pizza

On Friday night my husband and I took a break from the Meltdown work and went out to eat at a local pizza restaurant. Just as I was about to help myself to a second slice, a woman slid into the booth right next to me.

"Don't even think about eating a second piece," she ordered. I looked at this stranger who was interfering with my stolen pleasure.

"Hi," she said, finally introducing herself. "I'm Kathy Palmer, your neighbor."

I put down the second piece—be serious when you go public with your commitments!—and before we finished eating, Kathy had become the designated captain of captains. She would gather the statistics from team leaders, send out weekly newsletters and updates, and write the Friday Meltdown report in the *Union*. Kathy's background in computers,

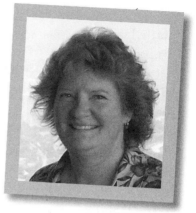

Kathy could have run the entire Roman Empire. Her organizational skills are extraordinary. As Captain of Captains, she keeps all of us on track.

her proximity (she lived across the street), her wonderful sense of humor, her writing skills, and her commitment to her own and others' fitness made her perfect for the job.

Spontaneous Creativity

The Meltdown had taken on a life of its own. Creative ideas for enhancing the program popped up everywhere. Prizes for individual and team achievements started coming in unsolicited. A cosmetics distributor donated beautiful product baskets. A manicurist donated manicures. A lifestyle counselor donated coaching. One dentist, in addition to donating fifteen teeth whitenings, offered a $10,000 dental makeover.

The evening programs also took on a life of their own. By the third meeting pre-event activities expanded spontaneously. Volunteers stood out front directing traffic in the chilly winter rain. Inside, other volunteers arranged chairs. Nurses were offering free blood pressure and body fat testing at one set of tables. One particularly devoted participant came early to decorate the stage, trucking in and arranging plants and silk trees.

Jazzercise instructors set up an aerobic program at the back of the huge hall. When participants, now dubbed "Meltdowners," walked in, they saw forty to fifty fitness buffs moving in orchestrated routines to energizing music—irresistible! Jazzercise devotees as well as people who had never tried dance as exercise joined in on the spot.

Nevada Irrigation District, the local water agency, provided free bottled water for meetings. Weight Watchers donated dozens of T-shirts for participants.

In another corner of the room, an expert in tai chi demonstrated with his apprentices. Staff from a massage school set up a worktable so participants could receive minimassages before and after the programs. To help the hearing impaired, a volunteer came forward to translate the program into sign language.

Members of teams showed up early to walk together around the perimeter of the room. I'd rarely seen such a festive atmosphere. People were laughing, cooperating, and celebrating. Political, religious, and economic divisions disappeared. We were working toward a common goal—helping each other get fit.

Don't Get Mad, Get Even!

With several hundred people engaged in dozens of different activities, neither Mike nor I noticed that a flyer had been placed on each chair, the same flyer we had found on our car windshields at the prior meeting. The flyer promoted an outrageously unsafe weight-loss product promising a quick fix.

What a wonderful experience it is to walk into the pavilion! Jazzercise students fill the air with their music and enthusiasm.

Strangers when they met, these women quickly become good friends.

Sharing our struggles and our successes cuts our burden in half and doubles our joy.

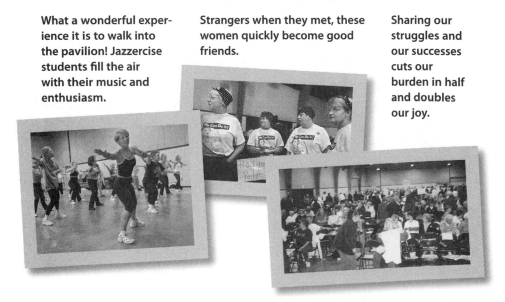

To make sure Meltdowners knew that this was not anything Mike and I had approved, I opened the evening's program by asking each person to stand up and wave the flyer over their head. Then I asked everyone to tear up every flyer in the room. Through this physical act, we were rejecting quick fixes and attempts to exploit us. The strategy worked. No one tried to take advantage of our program after that!

When we opened the mike to members of the audience, individuals shared their stories. Whether the week had stymied them or they'd made great progress, audience members always cheered them loudly.

Then individuals and teams who'd lost the most weight during the week were given special recognition. By then many teams wore matching costumes, some of them designed and made at home. We announced, among others, Just for the Health of It, Big Losers, Fast Women, Go Group Go, Gut Busters, Ten Percent Off, Half a Ton of Fun, and the Meltaways. People were having even more fun with their team names than their costumes!

During the open mike period, one young woman, Sirci Kitir, gingerly came up onstage on crutches. She told the audience about her ankle sprain, which she'd suffered just as the Meltdown was starting. Rather than miss out on the opportunity, she and her mother had decided to participate anyway. She was continuing her workout but was forced to limit herself to upper-body exercises. The crowd cheered her perseverance.

Another woman came up—Dena Nick, the stay-at-home mother of six. After deliberating long and hard about whether she would be taking time away from her family, she had finally decided to participate. When she talked about her commitment to her own fitness despite the pressures of raising a houseful of children, people erupted into wild applause.

Celebration Time, Come On!

There was much to celebrate. We now had 175 teams with 859 registered participants, and those numbers were, we knew, just the tip of the iceberg, since we had no way of counting all of the unofficial participants. Our total weight loss to date was approaching three thousand pounds—about a half a ton a week. Joking among ourselves, we boasted that we were becoming "weapons of mass reduction."

Medical Risks of Obesity

Amid our lightheartedness, we had serious business to attend to. Robin Wright Mallery, RN, was our guest speaker for the third meeting, and she talked about the medical risks of obesity and lack of fitness. From her role as coordinator for the hospital's cardiac rehabilitation center, Robin knew firsthand about the life-preserving importance of healthy habits, including regular exercise.

She explained the connection that researchers have found between lifestyle choices—eating and drinking too much, smoking, too little sleep and exercise—and serious medical conditions. Carrying extra weight makes the heart work harder to supply blood through the arteries and veins to the additional fat, she told us. The additional work raises blood pressure. Fifty million Americans, about one in five, have high blood pressure, and of the millions who have it, only one person in four has well-controlled blood pressure. Overweight people are also less efficient in metabolizing fat, which results in an increased blood level of LDL, the "bad" cholesterol linked to coronary heart disease.

Treat Health Problems? Treat Lifestyle

Treatment for heart disease, Robin told us, focuses first on changing lifestyle. Giving up smoking, losing weight, increasing exercise, choosing nutritional foods, and managing stress are the first lines of defense. Such is also the case with high blood pressure and Type II diabetes, other serious conditions that can be triggered by extra weight: a healthier lifestyle is the first line of treatment.

The risk of all the conditions related to obesity—stroke, breast and colon cancer, sleep apnea, gall bladder ailments, depression, gastric reflux disease, women's reproductive disorders—can be reduced through losing weight. The solution is as simple to do as it is difficult to achieve: bring food consumption into alignment with caloric expenditure and exercise to boost metabolism and maintain vitality. In other words, eat only what you can burn, and through exercise burn everything you eat.

Participants swarmed around Robin after her presentation. Despite our laughter and high spirits, we were all taking the medical implications seriously.

Helping Each Other Make Changes

Before the evening ended a dietitian at the hospital offered a free class to participants on nutrition, calories, and cooking styles. When we asked how many would show up for the weekly community walk, more hands went up than the week before. A second group announced their Saturday morning walks at the fairgrounds. New friendships were blossoming as people gathered for these community events.

We were discovering that becoming fit together would involve every part of us. To make positive changes, we needed to contribute all we had—our participation, enthusiasm, talents, and expertise.

Teaming Up for Friendship

Here we were in our third week, still adding new teams to the roster. Moreover, teams that had formed as a result of the Meltdown were turning our community not only into the fittest little county but also the friendliest. Some teams were made up of people who knew each other: coworkers formed teams from local banks, the community hospital, the local newspaper, a beauty salon, the school bus company, and a lumberyard. Two Methodist churches, from Grass Valley and Nevada City, challenged each other.

Most teams, though, were composed of complete strangers who had met at the first week's event and were now in the process of becoming friends. Backgrounds and professions varied. Losing in Style Team 1, by the end one of the most successful groups, was composed of a retired deputy sheriff, a stay-at-home mom, a highway patrol officer, a bank manager, a diesel mechanic, and a manicurist. Ages varied from our oldest citizen, eighty-year-old Carolyn Glithero, to teenage girls from the Friendship Club, an advocacy group for girls. Women outnumbered men about four to one. The mix was energizing.

Already some groups were thinking into the future. One group was planning the extension of their group effort into the spring. Other teams that did not want to be part of the "official" stats were nonetheless participating. One such husband, wife, and married daughter formed a threesome team. They began sharing and rating recipes, cooking together, and cheering each other on. This family unit assured me that their efforts would not end when the program ended.

Shifting Priorities

My days evolved into a blur of activity, beginning as early as I could rise and ending when I had not an ounce of energy left. The laundry piled up and meals became less organized. With a fitness club to run and hundreds of new clients to absorb, Mike's schedule was as demanding as mine. Thankfully, we'd set things up to be efficient: our phone calls and e-mails, though friendly, were exquisitely brief.

I was determined to keep my eating and exercise regimen, but something had to go. The momentum of the Meltdown was continuing to build, and there was no way I could skip town now. With a pang of loss, I realized that my long-awaited vacation in Kauai would become the first casualty. I dreaded telling my husband, since we had bought nonrefundable tickets and prepaid the condominium.

I was sorry to lose the vacation, but in its place I was gaining the joy that participants were communicating. Every day I received phone calls, e-mails, and letters from people excited by the results they were achieving.

Tears of Joy

One woman called in tears—tears of joy!—because for the first time in years, after losing weight and exercising during the Meltdown, she could touch her toes. She could even, she said, sleep on her stomach. She was thrilled.

Another participant, Jeannie Moore, the owner of Charlie's Angels Café, called to get help designing a special menu for Meltdowners. A participant herself, she said she looked around the room during the weekly meeting and saw many people who were her customers. I put her in touch with the hospital dietitian, and within a week Jeannie had introduced a new Meltdown menu, one that was instantly popular.

A half-dozen restaurants quickly followed suit. The grocery store chain SPD offered Meltdown recipes in its produce department. The owner of a motel, Courtyard Suites, charted out a mile-long walk through downtown Grass Valley and then arranged for a discount on meals at Charlie's Angels Café as a reward for completing the trek.

Sierra Nevada Memorial Hospital's cafeteria began offering a special menu for staff and visitors featuring Meltdown-friendly choices. A local kitchen supply store, Tess' Great Kitchen Place, offered specials on utensils, like a steamer, that could be used to prepare lower-calorie meals.

Mill Street Clothing, a prominent women's clothing store, offered discounts to participants who were steadily shrinking and could use the lift of new, smaller-sized clothes.

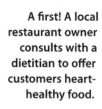

A first! A local restaurant owner consults with a dietitian to offer customers heart-healthy food.

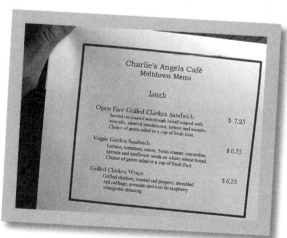

Like a pebble thrown into a pond, the circle of influence kept expanding.

The Meltdown had brought together people from all walks of life. Politics, religion, age, and wealth didn't matter. People and businesses were contributing imagination and creativity to the Meltdown in ways that I never could have imagined. We were coming together as a community.

I was tired at the end of each day, but my spirits were always lifted by the unfolding events. Mike and I were no longer in charge of the Meltdown; the Meltdown was in charge of us.

Beaming Our Message Beyond

Let your light shine—shine within you
so that it can shine on someone else.
Let your light shine.

OPRAH WINFREY

Thanks to the speed of today's communications, our community's effort to shape up was spreading beyond Nevada County, even beyond California. Through e-mail, participants were sharing their Meltdown experience with family members all over the United States. The *San Francisco Chronicle*, *San Jose Mercury News*, and *Sacramento Bee* newspapers printed articles on the developing event.

Traveling in South Africa, one local resident was amazed to read about the Meltdown in the *Argus*, a Capetown newspaper. Evidently the article written by Eric Bailey, the *Los Angeles Times* reporter who'd attended the second meeting, had been picked up by the Associated Press and reprinted in English-speaking papers worldwide.

My college roommate called from Chicago to let me know that her friends were all abuzz about the Meltdown. The *Chicago Tribune* had carried the story.

Two days later Dave and Rona, a well-known husband-and-wife radio personality team broadcasting on ABC's WLS, called for an interview. Both avid fitness advocates, they were enthusiastic about the Meltdown, and their relaxed style helped me forget that our conversation was reaching listeners in eight states.

Five Sacramento television stations regularly covered our progress on the evening news. *NewsTalk Radio* in Sacramento also wanted an interview, along with KGO Radio in San Francisco. Addresses on e-mails I was receiving indicated people from around the United States were tracking our progress. They wanted either advice for themselves or help in getting their own community Meltdowns started.

One Giant Leap

Arriving home late Thursday afternoon, I heard my husband ask if I knew Katie Couric. The name was vaguely familiar. I thought about everyone I played tennis with but couldn't remember anyone by that name. Maybe, I thought, she was one of the Meltdown team captains.

"Nope," I replied.

"The *Today* show," he prompted. He paused, then added nonchalantly, "She wants you to call her back."

I stood quietly in my kitchen. Time seemed to stand still beside me. In that moment I became aware and in awe of the mysterious way my personal distress and misery had been transformed into a force for good.

In the next moment, back to my practical self, I tried to figure out how to respond. I was up to my eyeballs in producing each week's event and still committed to exercising each day; I had precious little time to deal

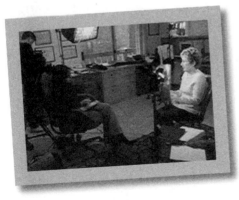

I worried that I'd be tongue-tied during my television interview at home. Once the interview begins, I forget to be nervous—I have so much to say!

with the media. The current week's project was to get "Ask Me about the Meltdown" buttons ordered and delivered in time for the Tuesday meeting so Meltdowners could start wearing them during the week.

Mike and managers of the other fitness clubs were equally busy absorbing hundreds of new members into their clubs. We had given out at least a thousand passes by this time. But we knew that if we wanted other communities to replicate our experience, we had to respond to the media.

Help!

I made a quick call to my son Marc. He recommended we get professional advice from his friend Jillian Elliott, a public relations specialist. I called Jillian and was delighted when she picked up the phone.

"Tell me what to do about this Katie Couric phone call," I pleaded.

"Call the number they left with your husband," she responded calmly. "You'll probably talk to a producer. Give them my name and number, and I'll take it from there." She added, "You might start thinking about people who can join you on the show. Get a representative group."

Jillian's calm and familiarity with the process were reassuring. I quickly made the call and passed along the contact information, then returned to planning the next event and the new task of lining up Meltdowners for the *Today* show.

Jillian had the job of coaching inexperienced, ill-prepared, and in some cases reluctant individuals for the glare of a national spotlight. From names I gave her, she quickly put together a representative group—the mayor of Nevada City, a beauty salon owner, a newspaper columnist, the mother of six who now was an enthusiastic participant, the Nevada City Methodist Church pastor, the owner of a restaurant, a manicurist, the young mother with a sprained ankle, and an elementary school teacher. Each had a unique perspective.

A Truck the Size of Utah

On Tuesday the NBC crew and transmitting truck arrived in Grass Valley. The huge semi moved slowly through the lightly falling snow and up the narrow mountain road to my home, where the show would be taped early the following morning. Once the truck driver arrived, he couldn't get the rig into the driveway.

The phone rang at our home. "I've got a truck out here the size of Utah," the driver told my husband. I looked out my office window and laughed at the monstrous truck blocking the road. "There's no way I can get in. What's the next plan?" he asked good-naturedly.

We hastily made arrangements to broadcast the following morning from Courtyard Suites, a new motel in town. Later I learned that heads had turned as the truck moved slowly through the narrow city streets of Grass Valley on its way to the motel.

Maybe I Should Watch More Television!

Right before I left for the Meltdown meeting that night, I made the mistake of checking my e-mail. There was a brief message from a producer from MSNBC's *Countdown with Keith Olbermann*. They wanted to do a segment on the Meltdown and asked me to call.

I was both delighted and overwhelmed. We hadn't even done the *Today* show yet, and we needed to prepare for another national network show! I called Jillian and said the magic word: "Help!"

She asked me to forward the request to her. "Not to worry," she added. "I'll work out the details and get back to you."

The Fourth Meeting Begins Earlier Than Ever

Despite the snowstorm, participants arrived at the fourth meeting earlier than they had the week before. Parking was now at a premium due to the crowds, and seats filled quickly.

After participants were greeted by volunteers at the door, they quickly became part of the buzz of voices, music, and movement throughout the hall.

Several hundred people were Jazzercising, talking, walking laps, buying buttons, getting their blood pressure checked, weighing in, sharing the results of the week with teammates, receiving messages, practicing tai chi, or getting massages. The number and variety of pre-event activities

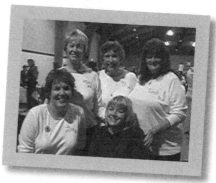

Here's a team of newfound friends cheering each other on.

kept increasing. We seemed to love the time we spent together playing before the program began.

As our weight loss was accumulating, we struggled with how to make the numbers meaningful. Fred Lossman, the volunteer coordinator, along with fellow car buffs, had planned a special event for this night to demonstrate visually what three thousand pounds looks like.

When the giant doors at the rear of the exhibit hall opened, everyone stood and turned around, delighted. Cheers, whistles, shouts, and clapping accompanied a decorated VW Beetle on its way to the front of the room, where the mayor of Nevada City, now a dedicated Meltdowner, got out. He and the VW together weighed 2,480 pounds.

Already the numbers were obsolete. By the time all the weight losses were reported for the evening, we realized we had lost two tons of fat, over four thousand pounds.

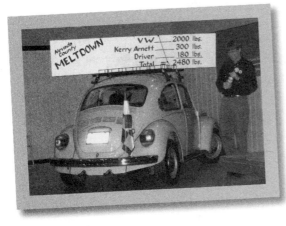

Seeing is believing! The VW gives us a tangible way to comprehend how many pounds we had lost.

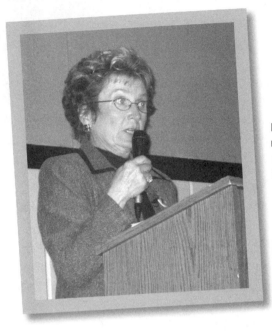

Each time I teach, I try to express myself in ways that have genuine meaning and impact, with words that ring true for participants.

Once the laughter and applause subsided, we took up a more serious matter—the problem of exercising and injuries. Because we knew John Seivert's reputation as an outstanding physical therapist, we had asked him to present information on how to avoid injuries.

A graduate of Northern Arizona University, John had earlier completed two postgraduate degrees in Australia. As a fellow of the American Academy of Orthopaedic Manual Physical Therapists (AAOMPT) and a member of the American Physical Therapy Association (APTA) and the National Strength & Conditioning Association (NSCA), John was well recognized in his field. Since 1991 he had regularly taught manual therapy courses to physicians and other medical professionals locally and nationally.

Beyond his qualifications, though, I had personal reasons to appreciate his expertise. A few years earlier, I had experienced excruciating pain in my back so that I could barely dress myself. Instead of prescribing a lifetime supply of Vicodin, my doctor sent me to John. The next day, John had me out playing tennis—granted, for only five minutes, but it was a start. John assured me—and I found it to be true—that if I conscientiously performed his prescribed back exercises each day, I could move entirely pain free.

Maintaining an Exercise Program Without Injuring Your Back

John had a kid's enthusiasm for life and was a competitive triathlete and bike racer. No wonder his first advice to us was to "play regularly." He said we'd find the right exercise because doing it would elicit uncontrollable smiles, fits of laughter, and childlike behavior. "Before you know it," he assured, "you'll become more fit than you ever dreamed possible, whatever your age." At the same time, he cautioned us to find an exercise appropriate for our body condition and age.

Core strength is crucial, John said, because "the most common problem in my practice is low back pain, a condition that affects over 80 percent of the population." While it was reassuring to know that most people recover from an acute episode within four to six weeks, he warned us that there's an 80 percent chance of recurrence within the next twelve months, especially if the underlying cause isn't corrected. He recommended a daily routine to develop core strength (comparable to brushing one's teeth for dental hygiene), which could be designed with professional guidance. Good posture at work and play was essential to reduce the chance of injury.

Knowing that many of us would be tempted to shift responsibility to our doctors and physical therapists to take away our pain, John ended his presentation by telling us that each one of us must take personal responsibility for the care of our bodies and especially our backs. He offered Meltdown participants free classes at his facility, and immediately a line of people formed to sign up.

Why Were We Getting National Attention?

I closed the evening by asking what made the Meltdown special. Why were we receiving so much national attention? After reflecting on this completely unexpected development, I'd concluded it was because we were ordinary people doing something extraordinary. In fact, I'd ordered T-shirts that said, "Ordinary People Doing Extraordinary Things." Meltdowners could purchase as many as they wanted at cost. At the end of the program the shirts flew out of the boxes as fast as we could unpack them. Some participants immediately put them on over their clothes. Through the T-shirts and the "Ask Me about the Meltdown" buttons, we had become walking advertisements for fitness.

Finally back home, I made last-minute phone calls to everyone appearing on the *Today* show to make sure they knew about the change of venue. I finished my final call about midnight and tumbled into bed for three hours of sleep.

Wide-eyed in the dark, I tried to not think about the number of people who would be watching. The thought was terrifying. Instead, I visualized I would be talking just to one person, Katie Couric. I fell asleep praying for guidance and the right words.

From Fat City to Tiny Town

We don't know who we are until we see what we can do.
MARTHA GRIMES

The alarm was set for 3:00 AM, but we didn't need it since we were both awake when it went off. We headed to the motel at 4:00 in order to broadcast live at 5:00 (8:00 in New York).

Rain was drizzling lightly. The transmitting equipment on top of the semi across the street from the motel was impressive even in the darkness. Trying to keep my hair from getting soggy, I dashed for the suite NBC had rented. My husband followed, carrying a bag of background materials we'd need to review before the show. Baby butterflies flitted in my stomach as I climbed a flight of stairs.

The women darted nervously in and out of the single bathroom, checking hair and makeup one last time. Fortunately, one participant was a hairstylist, another a makeup artist. We kept both busy wanting to look our best for our debut on national television.

Gingerly we took our places in the living room of the motel suite, trying not to trip on the many cables crisscrossing the carpeted floor. The local producer arranged our placements and gave instructions to the technicians for hooking up the body microphones.

At last we were seated and miked. The producer gave us last-minute instructions, reviewing once again the format for the show. She also alerted us to the one- to two-second delay in transmission, the time it would take for Katie Couric's signal to travel across the country to the West Coast. With about ten minutes to go, she called the producer in New York on her cell phone. We sat and listened raptly but understood nothing of their technological jargon. Anxiously, we waited for our next cue.

The moments before we went live were much worse than the actual interview. Once on the air, we responded to Katie Couric and Matt Lauer's questions as directly and briefly as we could. Matt and Katie asked me first about my own fitness makeover and how the Meltdown had come into existence. Then Ranee Lawson, captain of two teams called Losing in Style I and Losing in Style II, shared her enthusiasm and the support she felt at work and even from strangers when shopping for groceries. Jerry Smith, pastor at the Nevada City Methodist Church, joked about the competition between his church and a church in Grass Valley where his wife, Barbara Smith, serves as pastor. Lastly, Jeannie

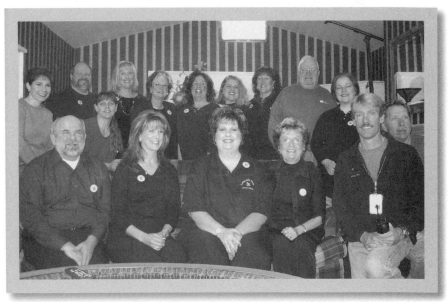

Until the last moment, the scene is chaotic. Then we wait for the show to begin. Except for the sound of rain outside, the room is tensely silent. I am eager to get the event behind me.

Moore talked about creating the new Meltdown menu in her restaurant, Charlie's Angels Café.

The interview time went by so quickly that we were surprised when it ended, even as we heaved a collective sigh of relief. Jillian had coached us well.

We celebrated with a breakfast at Charlie's Angels Café. Because of the three-hour delay in broadcasting on the West Coast, we had plenty of time to congratulate each other and still be home in time to watch our debut.

The Family Report Comes In: Two Thumbs Up!

Like everyone else in the group, I had alerted family and friends throughout the United States so that they could watch the show at their local time. My mother and sister Kay, in Iowa, saw the show two hours before I did. Kay said she thought I looked a little nervous. Since I was a lot nervous, I considered it a compliment. Overall they gave us a thumbs-up. Now I could relax when the program was finally shown in California.

After we watched the program and high-fived everyone in sight, I gave in to fatigue and crawled into bed for a rare midday nap. I had slept for only an hour when the phone woke me. It was Jillian. She'd been in touch with the producer from MSNBC. Here we go again!

The crew planned to tape a segment, and Jillian had already made the arrangements; all I had to do was to give an interview at home later that afternoon. I scrambled to get dressed and straighten my office. Already in Grass Valley, the crew was interviewing people in fitness centers, in restaurants, and on the street. My interview, later in the afternoon, went smoothly, considering how quickly events were occurring.

The Fittest Little County in the Nation

The next night, Thursday, *Countdown with Keith Olbermann* on MSNBC aired the segment called "Fat City, USA, Trying to Become Tiny Town." I didn't mind the good-natured teasing our community received. After all, we might be a little overweight, but we were at least working as a community to get fit. Would others do the same?

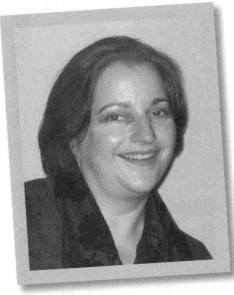

Jillian is a master at meeting publicity demands. Undaunted, she takes all requests and makes arrangements for interviews without missing a beat. Aren't we fortunate to have her?

We relished the opportunity to set an example and encourage other communities to undertake similar programs. We had set our goal to become the fittest little county in the nation, and we challenged other communities to beat our record.

At the same time, we realized that people everywhere in this country have in their hearts the desire to become fit and lose weight. We were no heavier than people elsewhere in the nation; we were just willing to admit our problem and start working on it.

Snow Falls on Our Fifth Meeting

We were now entering the fifth week of the program. Snow was falling, but the winter storm didn't keep participants away or dampen our enthusiasm that night. This time the West Coast office of CBS had sent a crew. They'd spent the day interviewing local people and attended the event that evening.

We began the evening by announcing our amazing results: to date, we had lost 4,978 pounds of fat, almost two and a half tons. At least two hundred teams and over a thousand people were officially participating. Many, many more people were informally involved, some in support of family members. Yet despite the hundreds of people present, our meetings felt like an intimate gathering among good friends.

This evening during the open mike time, one woman told of being able to reduce her blood pressure medication since starting the Meltdown. Others were striving for strength and balance. One woman told of being able to tie her shoes without her husband's help. Hearing their stories made the importance of fitness come alive. It wasn't an abstract concept—it affected all of us moment to moment each day.

Nothing was more central to the success of Meltdowners in achieving fitness than the decisions about food. We were actively discouraging members from trying to reduce their weight through dieting. In place

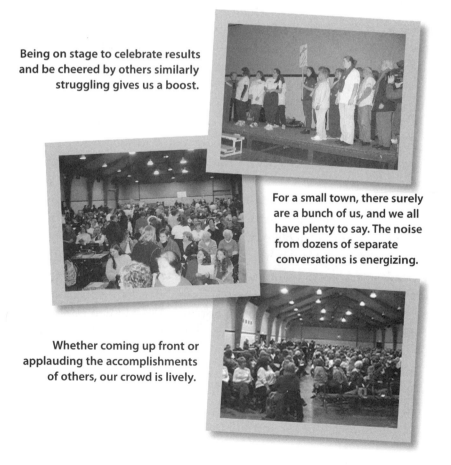

Being on stage to celebrate results and be cheered by others similarly struggling gives us a boost.

For a small town, there surely are a bunch of us, and we all have plenty to say. The noise from dozens of separate conversations is energizing.

Whether coming up front or applauding the accomplishments of others, our crowd is lively.

of dieting, we were promoting healthful eating, with weight loss being a happy by-product.

To explain healthful eating, Laura Seeman, a registered dietitian from Sierra Nevada Memorial Hospital, took the stage with a presentation not only humorous and articulate but also practical. Like the rest of us, she had struggled to realize her own weight goals.

Healthful Eating in a Nutshell

Her goal, Laura said, was to give us the five basics of healthful eating in a nutshell so we could reach and maintain our desired weight and level of fitness.

First, she said, forget dieting. Instead, commit to making permanent changes in lifestyle. Our aim would be to balance food choices over time so that we take in no more than we expend. For most of us, exercise and record keeping would help us realize long-term success.

Second, we should focus, she said, on the complex carbohydrates like whole grains, beans, fruits, and vegetables, which provide the body with energy. Avoid the simple carbohydrates found in candy, cookies, juice, and table sugar.

Third, she warned us that while protein is needed for growth and repair, it is not usually needed in the quantities commonly consumed. And, she added, when choosing, pick lean meats (white meat poultry and fish) and meat substitutes (cottage cheese and egg whites).

Fourth, we needed to learn to distinguish between fats—between the "good fats," found in olive oil, canola oil, peanut butter, and avocado, which are the best for the heart, and the less-healthy saturated fats in butter, dairy products, coconut, and chocolate. Watch out for trans fats, she warned us (partially hydrogenated oils found in some margarine, snack foods, crackers, and cookies), since they raise the bad cholesterol.

Fifth, Laura emphasized the importance of making better choices. Although many resources could help, she suggested a new book by Dr. Howard Shapiro, *Picture Perfect Weight Loss*. She found her clients could easily relate to the material in Dr. Shapiro's book because it contained visual comparisons on food choices, thereby demonstrating how we could eat more and better and still lose weight.

Because few topics are more emotionally complex and controversial than what we eat, participants flooded Laura with their questions. She responded by offering a free nutrition counseling class at the hospital.

Where Do I Find Time for My Own Exercise?

Giving radio interviews at odd hours, taping television segments at the request of various stations, and writing for the newspaper made time for my own exercise increasingly scarce. Jillian's solution was as simple as it was obvious: television segments would be taped during my actual workouts, either on the tennis court or in a fitness center, thereby accomplishing both goals at once.

It became necessary for Mike and me to work even more efficiently. Our e-mails were brief and our phone calls even briefer. The excitement of our jointly conceived project kept us from complaining about the workload and pressure. It also kept us from looking up from the row we were hoeing; we had just a few more weeks to go!

Resigned to the fact that we would not make it to Kauai, my husband continued to provide good-natured support. He eased my fears when an anxiety attack would strike in the middle of the night, and he also

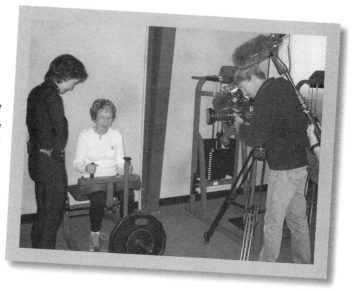

Maybe it isn't my regular workout, but at least I get some exercise.

handled household duties and ran errands for the Meltdown. His support was invaluable.

On those rare occasions when I did get into town, "Ask Me about the Meltdown" buttons appeared on coats and jackets almost everywhere. Sometimes I'd see a group of people walking together, proudly wearing their buttons and Meltdown T-shirts. I couldn't resist opening the window and chatting for a few minutes with these strangers. Hearing how excited they were about their progress—whether it was a woman who had gone down a dress size or people who found that they loved their morning walks—never failed to energize me.

) WEEK 6 (

The Tail Wags the Dog

Hell, there are no rules here—
we're trying to accomplish something.

THOMAS A. EDISON

Our e-mail network of designated point people for the various assignments was working efficiently. We were functioning professionally and reliably, yet all of us were volunteers stealing bits and pieces of time from other commitments, and we weren't always sure we knew what we were doing.

Even though we were in week six, more people were joining teams and more teams were filling our roster. New prizes kept coming in; more businesses were getting involved by offering discounted services or special bonuses to Meltdown participants. The chamber of commerce began promoting our commitment to fitness as an added bonus for living and working in the area. A social worker offered free weight counseling to participants. A Pilates studio offered free classes.

At our sixth meeting I announced our total weight loss: 204 teams with 1,032 participants had lost 5,856 pounds—almost three tons! One five-person team had lost over 70 pounds.

Though we had given out hundreds of free passes, Mike and I knew that some people would prefer to work out at home. For that reason we had invited Scott Jackson as our guest speaker to address issues involved in building your own home gym. Scott had an extensive background as a personal trainer and educator, and he owned a workout center, Real Life Fitness. Moreover, he could speak from experience: he had used exercise and sports as a way to control his own weight.

Creating Your Own Home Gym

Exercising at home, Scott said, is a good alternative for the person who is short on time, has home obligations or restrictions, or wants to work out in private. But, he cautioned, it's important to pick our fitness and health goals before purchasing equipment, as well as to think about whether our temperament lends itself to solo workouts.

At the practical level, before creating a home gym we must consider the equipment we already have at home, space available, space that will be needed, budget, and other family members' use of the equipment. Because answering these questions ahead of time can prevent expensive mistakes, he also suggested we get professional guidance from a qualified fitness consultant for both selecting equipment and choosing a gym routine.

Scott's obvious expertise triggered questions from dozens of people, and after the session ended he stayed and talked with them until volunteers had stacked the chairs and we were ready to lock up the hall for the night.

As Dick and I drove into our darkened driveway at midnight, I heaved a sigh of relief. Only two more meetings to go!

Ever the Pessimist—Participation Will Decline!

Each time I finished a session, I went home thinking that future attendance would probably decline. By now people would be getting the idea that fitness couldn't be achieved with a quick fix but rather involved a lifetime commitment. Surely that would kill off enthusiasm. And if having to think in years instead of weeks didn't do it, the winter rains and snows surely would.

But each week, instead of facing declining attendance, we were adding new members and additional teams. Fitness centers reported that more, not fewer, people were coming in to work out.

More media were contacting us. When CNN *Headline News* picked up a segment on the Meltdown story and televised it both nationally and internationally, we knew we were up to important work. What we were accomplishing was changing our own lives, but it was also affecting communities across the nation and around the world. Only when my son Steve, in France, caught the segment on the international version of CNN *Headline News* did the full import of what our community was doing hit him.

My three teenage granddaughters, in Missouri, accidentally saw a segment on the Meltdown on their local television station. "That's Grandma!" the youngest, Danielle, exclaimed.

They cheered in unison: "Go, Granny, go!"

On Sunday a special feature in the *Sacramento Bee* featured the Meltdown. The *Bee*'s status as the major newspaper in the state's capital meant that the article was noticed by residents throughout the state. Our small community, located seventy miles away from Sacramento in another county, wasn't used to the limelight, at least not unless a murder

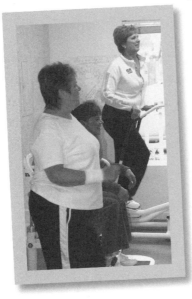

Making new friends
while exercising is
a big part of the fun.

had been committed (so rare it always made news). We were delighted to be the subject of a positive story this time, one that would energize rather than depress readers. We were the happy tail wagging the dog for a change!

A Lid for Every Pot

I've been on a diet for two weeks,
and all I've lost is two weeks.
TOTIE FIELDS

By now the outline of events for Tuesday night had evolved into a ritual that we all looked forward to. First we'd celebrate our results, individual and team, both for the prior week and for the Meltdown to date. Then we'd pass the microphone around or bring Meltdowners up on stage to tell about their successes and triumphs.

Because I was also working on the eighth and final event, I kept the program for the seventh meeting as simple and uncomplicated as possible.

Or at least I tried to.

My phone had rung the previous Sunday afternoon. The woman's name didn't stick, but her request did. She wanted to come onstage Tuesday night and perform a striptease. I listened for an opening so I could gently let her know that doing a strip show probably wouldn't work out.

Sensing my lack of enthusiasm, she hurried on. "You don't understand," she said. "I've gone through so many sizes of clothes as I've lost weight that I thought it would be fun to wear all of them, starting with my fattest clothes, and then peel them off one at a time until I'm down to the real me!" She added, "I'll bring my own music. You know the song they always play when a stripper takes her clothes off?"

I could picture her onstage as soon as she described it. It was a wonderfully creative way to show the impact of her fitness efforts.

Since we'd never met, I told her to check in with me at the start of the evening and I'd work her "stripping show" into the program. By now I felt like Ed Sullivan orchestrating an evening's worth of variety acts.

We Are Still Adding Teams

At our seventh meeting on yet another wet, cold, stormy night, we celebrated even more progress. Because people were still joining (our official registration was 1,048 and climbing), we were adding yet more teams. We were also continuing to average a weight loss of about a half a ton a week, an announcement that never failed to bring the house down.

Community members continued to offer their contributions. One person had posted twenty-two area hiking trails on the Meltdown Web site. In an effort to encourage people to get outdoors and walk, she had included the length, difficulty, and location of each hike—a valuable piece of research.

And more prizes continued to flow in. I took the time at our meeting to read the growing list. Not a single one had been solicited; all came spontaneously in support of what the Meltdowners were trying to achieve. Although there was genuine appreciation for the prizes, the real gift was the one participants were giving themselves— healthier bodies.

Then I introduced our stripper. "In the first session," I said, "Mike and I promoted the idea that exercise comes in many forms. We urged participants to find an exercise that they loved to do because they will be more likely to continue.

"One of them," I suggested, tongue-in-check, "might be developing a strip act. Dancing around a room could burn calories," I added. The audience looked puzzled, as if I had finally gone over the edge.

"With us tonight," I announced—now I was really Ed Sullivan!—"is a woman who will demonstrate this form of exercise." More puzzled looks. "She is going to demonstrate," I continued, "how much her body has shrunk as she has lost weight and gained fitness."

My stripper came on stage, bulked up in multiple layers of clothes. With the traditional stripping music blasting away, she proceeded to take off her first layer. Whistling and cheering, Meltdowners immediately got into the act. It was hard to tell whether the women or men were enjoying it more. It took only minutes before our stripper was revealing her current body—in a tight-fitting outfit. When she finished, everyone cheered loudly. We admired her courage in "stripping" in front of a thousand people and also her achievement in losing weight.

Baby Llamas Become Our Mascot

Still on a playful note, I reported on yet another unconventional form of exercise. In the second week of the Meltdown, it had been announced that Lorene Grassick, the owner of Highland Llama Trekkers, wanted volunteers to train her baby llamas. Lorene provided adult llamas to hikers, who used them to pack supplies.

The baby llamas needed to become comfortable with people and to get used to carrying packs. Lorene had noticed that the people who regularly walked the baby llamas trimmed down. So, she thought, why not offer this as an exercise to Meltdowners? They could enjoy the companionship of the sweet baby llamas and also the scenic trails and

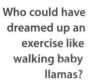
Who could have dreamed up an exercise like walking baby llamas?

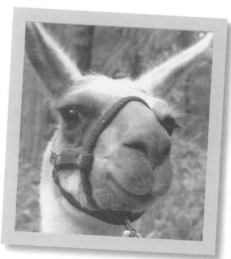

hiking paths in our section of the Sierra foothills. As a by-product, they'd trim down from the exercise.

Two weeks later I received an e-mail from Lorene. "We now have fifty people participating," she wrote. "Some to lose weight, some to gain strength and stamina, and some just for fun! Each one has a favorite llama to walk, and all are enjoying themselves. We go on a different trail each time, one weekend day and one weekday each week."

Talk about a lid for every pot! I'd never seen "baby llama walking" listed in an exercise manual, but it was working just fine for those fifty people.

No Diets!

It seemed that we never made it through an evening without getting peppered with questions about dieting. What was the best diet? Did we recommend the Atkins diet? What were the medical problems associated with a high-protein diet? Did we recommend Dr. Peter Gott's "no sugar, no flour" diet? If a person limited their calories to fewer than a thousand a day, would that give their body what it needed nutritionally?

People often asked me what diet I had used to lose weight. When I responded that I ate everything in moderation and had no forbidden foods, I always saw the person's face fall. Instead of dieting, I volunteered, I was looking for a way that I could eat for the rest of my life. Too often, it seemed, the person was looking for one special way of eating—one set of rules that would make pounds disappear. Or a pill to pop that would make pounds melt away. Instead, I wanted to offer a different way of living.

To address questions of dieting and drugs from a medical perspective, we brought in a local physician and a nurse-practitioner to give our seventh presentation.

Dieting, Lifestyle Changes, and Medical Considerations

Dr. Roger Hicks, medical director of Yuba Docs, and Kitty Kelly, family nurse-practitioner, both recommended long-term solutions based on a balanced diet rather than quick fixes. They began by reviewing a few of the more popular diets. A low-carbohydrate diet, such as Atkins and South Beach, offered the advantage of a suppressed appetite, which meant that people didn't walk around feeling hungry. Some people could lose weight on these diets, especially if they were insulin sensitive or diabetic.

The downsides, they hastened to add, were many. The diet can induce dehydration and ketosis (a pathological accumulation in the body of ketone substances). The immune system can also become suppressed. Other possible negatives include bruising, nausea, headache, dizziness, irritability, bad breath, disruption of sleep, and decreased exercise tolerance. Some patients also experienced gout, osteoporosis, elevated cholesterol, and coronary artery disease.

Moving on to the focused food diets (grapefruit diet, cabbage soup diet, chocolate diet, beer diet), our medical experts pointed out that these were really calorie-reduction diets because only selected foods are eaten. The downside, they added, was that boredom sets in and the dieter typically rebounds by eating more of the forbidden foods.

When it comes to the Atkins or South Beach or some other diet, our experts agreed, the net result is an imbalanced approach that leaves dieters feeling deprived. Plus, the special diet may cost more, nutritional deficiencies may occur, and blood sugar can be elevated.

Their strong recommendation: move into the "No Diet Zone." Instead of going on a diet, find the zone of permanent changes in nutrition and exercise and eating a wide array of colorful foods and vegetables. Stay in touch with your changing body, they suggested, so you can adjust your habits as your body develops and matures.

Depression is the most common cause of obesity, they said. Many people try to self-medicate for depression and anxiety by eating comfort foods, but this will only compound the problem. The real solution, they told us, is to treat the depression, since treating the depression may also boost weight loss.

Giving Up Magical Thinking

Our doctor and nurse-practitioner stripped away any illusions people may have had about quick-fix medical solutions to being overweight. "There are no magic pills to solve weight problems," Nurse Kelly said, "and surgery carries significant risks." Moreover, she added, surgery is typically limited to a person who is morbidly obese and has life-threatening weight problems. Even so, this person must demonstrate an ability to lose weight and willingness to undergo counseling. It is far more reasonable and practical to control weight before it gets to the point of obesity.

Their final recommendations took us back to the basics: stop dieting, start eating healthfully, and avoid fast food. If we must eat cookies, they said, make them from scratch by hand with no mixer! Any changes we make need to become permanent. To help us think about long-term goals, they asked, "What do you want to look like in ten years?" Once we knew the answer to this question, we could begin working today to reach that goal.

Their parting advice: "Lose the remote, exercise every day, walk up stairs when you get a chance, park as far away from the storefront as you can, and recruit family and friends to join you."

Llamas Lead the Way

At the conclusion of the program, the mayor of Nevada City, Kerry Arnett, invited Meltdowners to join the Mardi Gras parade in his town on Sunday. We decided that it was only fitting for the llamas to join us. With the mayor as our escort, about seventy of us paraded proudly through the streets, wearing our Meltdown buttons and T-shirts. Walking in our midst were a dozen llamas, who had come to symbolize our unique fitness project.

The Best Is Yet to Come!

*I get up every morning determined to both change the world
and have one hell of a good time.
Sometimes this makes planning my day difficult.*

E. B. WHITE

As soon as the seventh week's event was over, I began working with Mike on the last session. We had so much to accomplish in this final event, and we were determined to keep our promise to finish each session by 9:00.

And of course the producers at NBC's *Today* show with Katie Couric wanted to report to their viewers the final results of the Meltdown. The same group of media hounds would gather at the same motel. By now we knew the drill. The morning after the final event, we would need to set the alarm for 3:00, arrive at the motel by 4:00, broadcast at 5:00, and eat breakfast at 6:00. Then we'd go home to watch our presentation on television, along with the rest of the community and our families scattered throughout the United States.

More difficult to arrange was the taping of CBS's *The Early Show.* The producer wanted to broadcast the show live at the fairgrounds in the main hall—the large, cavernous room where all of our successes had been reported—but at 3:00 AM.

So much for the luxury of sleeping until three! My job was to persuade a supportive group of Meltdowners to crawl out of bed on a stormy night and come back to the fairgrounds at 2:30 AM for the broadcast. Good luck, I said to myself. If they do it, they're truly going above and beyond the call of duty.

I didn't have time to worry about the fact that once we finished with CBS, we'd have about twenty minutes to change clothes and race to the motel to begin taping the NBC show. Whenever I allowed myself to contemplate the coming events, my stomach did flip-flops. So I forced myself to focus instead on planning the final evening's event. My theory was that this would keep my mind off the impending media appearances. Fat chance!

Ultimately four television networks covered the final event, giving us opportunities to challenge communities throughout the United States to better our record. Until then, we would retain our self-proclaimed title as "the fittest little county in the nation."

Jillian was scrambling in her efforts to respond to the producers' requests. To expedite her work, she decided to camp out at my house for the final few days. I was delighted. She could help me pick clothes to wear—my wardrobe was still limited because of the weight I had lost—and also help me rehearse our message.

The Durham Dolls Ride in Style

Thanks to the help of one special team, the Durham Dolls, Mike and I had a fabulous final evening planned. These women drove school buses for the Durham Transportation Company, transporting students to and from our schools.

The team came up with the idea of opening the back doors of the exhibit hall during the event to depict the nearly four tons of weight (the amount we had lost) as realistically as possible. They had obtained permission from their employer to borrow a bus for the evening, and they had decorated it with hundreds of team names and many, many balloons. The bus sat at the ready, secretly parked in a hidden area behind huge hinged doors at the back of the hall.

The Big Finale

On the day of the final event, my eyes flew open at 5:00 AM; I wouldn't need an alarm clock today. Quietly slipping out of bed so I wouldn't disturb my husband, I headed to my office. A dozen or so urgent e-mails had to be sent to finalize details for tonight.

Mike and I were also scheduled to meet with the Nevada County Board of Supervisors at 9:00 AM. We would update them on the results of the proclamation they had issued at the start of the Meltdown. Was it really only seven weeks ago? It seemed now like the far distant past!

After seven weeks of hard work, Mike and I appreciated the opportunity to brag about the achievements of the individuals and teams as well as to commend the contributions of businesses and individuals in the community. We had so much to report. Not only had people in our community lost a total of four tons of excess weight, but between regional, national, and international coverage in print and on radio and television, we figured we had made a positive impact on millions, ordinary people who had learned that other ordinary people in Nevada County were successfully losing weight together.

The supervisors were pleased that their proclamation had contributed to the larger effort. Once again political differences dissolved as they commended the residents of the county for their remarkable achievement and also for the added bonus of a renewed sense of community.

I raced home from the supervisors' meeting to finish work on the evening's events. Emi was already fielding phone calls and responding to e-mails. It would be a busy day.

Largest Group Ever

Late that afternoon I arrived at the main gate to the fairgrounds. The parking lot was already a third full just with the cars of volunteers and early arrivals. Taking up a large portion of the parking lot was a huge semitruck with big letters, CBS, covering its side. Adjacent to the CBS truck were other television transmitting units. Thank goodness the NBC truck was located at the motel instead of here, or the Meltdowners wouldn't have had any place to park!

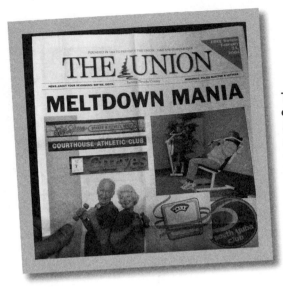

To celebrate our success, the *Union* published a special edition: "Meltdown Mania."

When about twelve hundred people arrived that night, they found a special edition of the *Union* on their chairs, honoring the Meltdown and the community support that had made it all possible. They made their way around the half-dozen television crews jockeying for positions to tape the evening's events. The Sacramento TV crews would cover the event live and feed their stories to their networks.

With one arm Jillian steered me to a few interviews and with the other arm pointed reporters to team members willing to share their success stories. I spent a few minutes with a reporter from the *Sacramento Bee* before I passed him along to an eager Meltdowner who soon passed him along to yet another person with an enthusiastic story to tell.

Celebration Time! Come On In and Join the Party!

As we had in the past, we started promptly at 7:00. The program began with four charming high school girls singing the national anthem a cappella to a respectful audience. Next high school music teacher Rod Baggett and his wife, Julie, led us in a Meltdown sing-along. The two had written knock-off lyrics for the Meltdown to the tune of *The Beverly Hillbillies*, the old television show theme. Laughing, the audience joined in.

The Meltdown Song

words by Rod and Julie Baggett

Stop and let me tell you about a little mountain town
They all came together just to drop tons of pounds
They broke up into teams, and became goal bound
They called themselves Nevada County Meltdown.

Carole Carson, visionary! Mike Carville, fitness expert!

The next thing they did was get off the easy chair
Threw out the junk food like donuts and éclairs
Put their tennis shoes on and started runnin' round the block
Before too long their muscles were hard as rock.

Treadmills, salads! Eight-minute abs, no liposuction!

As the weeks went along they were stepping on the scale
The pounds just dropped as they were workin' off their tail
They came to all the meetings, the momentum never died
They made national news and instilled some county pride.

Tom Brokaw, Katie Couric! Who needs Oprah and Dr. Phil?

Eight weeks later Meltdown is going strong
This is not a phase but a way to live life long
The people and the businesses in our community
All came together just to help you and me.

*Restaurants, exercise clubs, health professionals help trade those
pear shapes for hourglass figures!*

You just don't know but your life depends on it
Let's be fit and trim and never, ever quit
We're all in this together, so keep our spirits high
Just keep on exercising and reaching for the sky.

The laughing and applause finally wound down, and in that moment of silence came a blast of music over the loudspeakers while the rear doors of the auditorium carefully opened. A huge yellow school bus driven by the Durham Dolls slowly made its entrance. Covered with signs and decorated with balloons, the bus rolled by row after row of cheering Meltdowners.

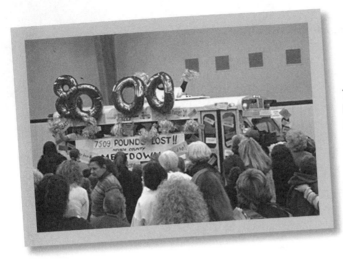

Through the open bus windows, the Dolls wave as the audience whistles, yells, and applauds.

Together, we'd lost 7,509 pounds of fat, the approximate weight of the bus and its passengers. The Durham Dolls had given tangible form to our jaw-dropping results. We cheered long and hard, bursting with pride at our accomplishment.

Then we passed out special prizes to the top-performing teams and gave away the remaining prizes. With so much community generosity, distributing prizes took almost half an hour.

We handed out *Take Five* cookbooks provided by Weight Watchers to each of the captains to thank them for keeping track of team members and faithfully reporting weight information. We thanked the fitness clubs for their generosity in donating more than 1,700 eight-week free passes. We thanked the volunteers working on the scene and behind the scene. We thanked the businesses who had created special offers and discounts for participants.

Just Beginning

The final, hearty thanks went to the group as a whole for its willingness to experiment in a community fitness project. We had not finished but were only beginning. But how far we had come in eight weeks! My dream was that each of them would continue and encourage others to join them.

We had undertaken our experiment trusting that we had the energy and commitment to bring something good to our lives and to each other. The future would determine the full implications for the Meltdowners, for our community, and for our neighbors elsewhere in the United States.

For many, the benefits of the lifestyle changes were real and immediate: reduced medications, especially for diabetics; lower blood pressure; improved outlook and appearance; more stamina and energy; improved self-esteem; and, for many of us, new friends. As real as those benefits were, we couldn't measure the number of heart attacks or strokes that had been prevented or delayed or how many additional years we had collectively added to the lives of Meltdowners.

At the beginning of the series I had stated with conviction that we had the resources to accomplish our task—to make ourselves "the fittest little county in the nation." We had the physical resources and a beautiful environment. We had the human resources and a wonderfully creative and generous community. And we had the vision.

Now I was more convinced than ever that we had a vitally important job to do. Our job was to be a catalyst not merely for ourselves and our own families but for others as well—for fellow students at school, for colleagues at work, and for members of our churches and social organizations. Although we were ending the Meltdown, I remained convinced that the best part was yet to come.

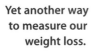

Yet another way to measure our weight loss.

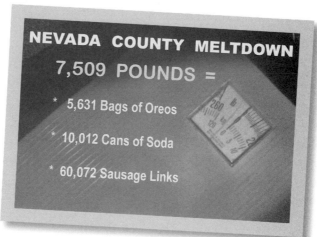

NEVADA COUNTY MELTDOWN
7,509 POUNDS =

* 5,631 Bags of Oreos
* 10,012 Cans of Soda
* 60,072 Sausage Links

Becoming a Catalyst for Others

After the exhilaration of the final evening, I found myself too excited to close my eyes. Setting the alarm for 2:00 AM, I enjoyed the quiet of my bedroom. I could hear the grandfather clock ticking downstairs.

Unable to sleep, I thought about the remarkable experience we'd just gone through, wondering where it would lead. Instead of counting sheep, I counted people who had contributed so much—Dick, Marc, Jillian, Mike, Emi, Kathy—the list went on and on.

Rain was falling when I turned off the alarm. Awake all night, I hadn't needed it.

To my surprise, several dozen people showed up for the 3:00 AM live CBS broadcast of *The Early Show*. All of us were still high from the prior night's event. The producer grouped us around the school bus—still parked and decorated in the pavilion from the night before. Despite blasts of heavy rain outside, the interview inside went smoothly. I challenged other communities to match or beat our record.

The minute the show was over, those scheduled to appear on the *Today* show ducked into restrooms. In the icy, unheated facilities, we quickly changed clothes and raced to the motel for our next appearance. During the second interview I repeated the challenge to other communities as I bragged about our almost four tons of lost weight.

Once again, the group celebrated with a breakfast at Charlie's Angels Café. Afterward, I went home to pack for my belated and

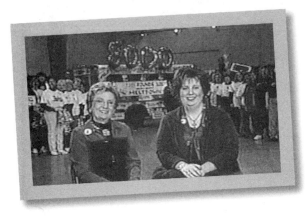

Despite the winter storm and fatigue, we are thrilled to be reporting our results to a national audience.

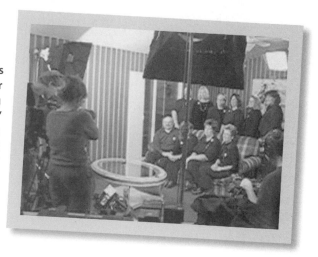

Deafening silence fills the room as we wait for our cue that we are going live. "Please, dear God," I pray, "make my heart stop pounding and tell me what to say!"

much-abbreviated trip to Kauai. My husband and I would take a few days to rest and finally enjoy unstructured time. Then I would see what the future held. I was absolutely certain that the best was yet to come.

For now, it was time to rest and recover.

A Community Comes Together

One person could not a Meltdown make. This event could not have happened without individuals, groups, and organizations taking personal responsibility for improving fitness. Sometimes their actions and support were public and visible; sometimes they were privately accomplished. A complete history of the Meltdown is nearly impossible to relate.

What we knew for certain, however, is that we were ordinary people doing an extraordinary thing, and we were doing it together.

) (

Getting off the Tiger
and onto a Bigger One

None of us will ever accomplish
anything excellent or commanding
except when he listens to this whisper
which is heard by him alone.
RALPH WALDO EMERSON

I used the ten days in Kauai to rejuvenate my marriage and gain perspective on what I had just been through. Relieved of the pressure of producing a weekly event, I luxuriated in sleeping late and squandering hours playing cards or reading a good mystery novel. I focused on getting back to an ongoing workout routine, indulging my passion for tennis in the early morning hours and later in the day when the ocean breeze had cooled the air.

I also used the time to reflect on my role and decide what the focus of my life would be now that the Meltdown was behind me. My guess was that I had ten to fifteen years of productive time left to live. How would I spend this precious time?

Retreat or Refocus? Step Down or Step Up?

Just as I had hoped others would step forward to lead the Meltdown, I now hoped that others in our community would step forward to take our results to a higher level. That didn't necessarily translate into another event.

My job as catalyst for the Meltdown was done. In the spotlight for eight weeks, I had planted seeds. Now it was time for others to pick up the seeds and plant them in their own universes—at work, in social clubs, in their religious organizations, in schools, and in their families. Only in this way could we realize the long-term benefits of our work; only in this way would the "best that was to come" materialize for us and our families.

Certainly I had personal business I wanted to attend to. Family obligations that had been put on hold during the Meltdown were mounting. Jamie, while continuing to make progress, still needed encouragement and support. Her children and other grandchildren were overdue for visits. My son and his wife in France were urging me to visit them.

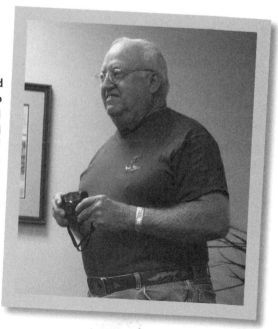

Here's Dick, my husband and one-man support team, who was always in the background and always ready to help. I had cheated him out of two weeks' vacation in Kauai. Maybe now we could spend more time together.

I wanted to continue to play on a tennis team, do some volunteer work, and spend time with my husband. I had shortchanged him on our trip to Kauai and wanted to make it up to him. When the people who rented the condominium learned why we had to give up a part of our vacation, they gave us credit for the unused time so we would be able to go back and play in Kauai at some future date.

I also wanted to get back to my sewing and quilting. Mike's baby girl had arrived, and I wanted to make her a nice baby quilt to thank him for his wonderful partnership. At last I could catch up!

Or could I?

I felt a nagging thought once again emerging. What about writing a book to share our experience with other communities?

I pushed the idea down, but it kept resurfacing.

And in addition to a book, what about a community television show to spotlight people who have made lifestyle changes? Many more people could be reached with the message of fitness, so what about speaking at community events?

I turned the thought off once again. I didn't have the resources to make all this happen. And for once I wanted to goof off!

But my protests were losing out. My vacation in Kauai wasn't even over, and already I knew I was going to have to get back on the tiger.

PART 4

Proliferating Weapons
of Mass Reduction

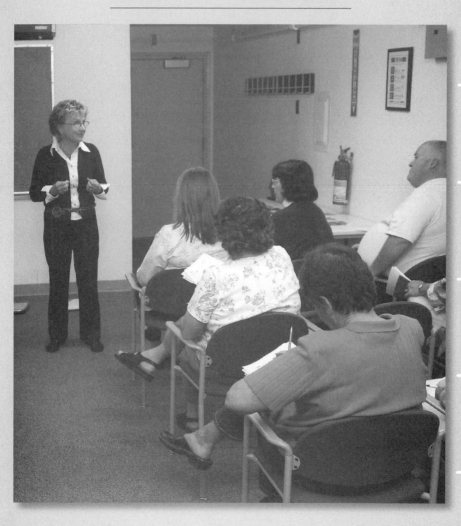

A ship in the harbor is safe—
but that is not what ships are built for.

LISA WILLIAMS

) (

I came home eager to begin the next phase, with dozens of ideas to promote fitness in our community and elsewhere. Some efforts might succeed, others fail. However they turned out, though, an ongoing effort to promote fitness would keep me honest—I'd have to set an example.

At the same time, I was sorry to leave Kauai behind after so short a visit. As eager as I was to get going, I recognized that I was giving up a leisurely retirement. I also worried about the added expenses. Maybe I should just return to my formerly private life instead of pursuing my fitness project.

I was at a crossroads. Either way would affect my marriage. I turned to my husband, Dick, for perspective.

"The extra expenses," he assured me, "will not be the issue." The money needed to pursue my volunteer work would not overwhelm us or require changes in how we lived. Always generous, he said he would consider the expenses a charitable contribution even if they weren't tax deductible.

But, critically important, he said, was reserving time together. He had been widowed at fifty-five when his wife died from colon cancer, and he didn't want our time together to slip away without his realizing his dreams of exploring new country. He was adamant that I preserve time for the two of us, especially time for car trips to national forests and parks.

I agreed, and I appreciated his understanding and unqualified support. Having worked through my concerns with Dick, I began allowing myself to envision even grander ways of promoting fitness.

In retrospect, I saw that this fork in the road was an illusion. The real fork in the road occurred the moment I stepped on the bath scale, it broke, and I decided to get fit. In an instant I went from recreational eater to nutrition nut and from quiet retiree to local columnist. Instead of moving into old age, I moved into a new stage. Everything else was flowing from this decision.

Although the view had changed, I was still on the same path. The new horizon was simply a function of the elevation I'd gained from continuing. It was time to take the message further, time to create an epidemic of fitness.

) (

Up Close and Personal: Getting Fit Together

*Friendship is born at that moment when one person
says to another: What! You too? I thought I was the only one.*

C. S. LEWIS

To figure out how to move forward, I needed to figure out where we'd
been. The obvious first step was to read the evaluations that had come
pouring in after the Meltdown.

The results were impressive. Although our community is small, 208
teams had registered, with a total of 1,058 participants. Many took part
for reasons unrelated to weight loss; even so, together we had shed a
grand total of 7,593 pounds.

A whopping majority felt they had improved their fitness. Half said
they had lost weight and had achieved sustainable lifestyle changes.
More than 80 percent said they would participate in future events.
Most amazingly, more than 40 percent of the team captains sent an
evaluation—a high rate of return.

The numbers were fun to brag about, but even more rewarding for
me personally was the sense of empowerment conveyed in what people
wrote. Dozens of letters spontaneously poured in. Individuals bragged
about their team's weight loss, as well as their own. They talked about the

impact their own changes were having on their families and friends. Others acknowledged the beginning of lifelong journeys toward better health.

The letters came from people at different stages of life and engaged in a variety of occupations—a teenager and an eighty-year-old, the mayor of Nevada City and a stay-at-home mom, a longtime resident and a new resident recently widowed and seeking friends, a beautician and a teacher. Overwhelmingly, their comments centered on one theme: liberation from personal, private shame and isolation.

The joy of being part of a team and larger community was expressed in dozens of ways. One participant wrote that the most important benefit for her was realizing that she didn't have to fight the battle alone. Another said that what made the difference for her was knowing that we were in this together.

Freely admitting problems with weight to others who were similarly struggling was a powerful experience. One woman wrote that she succeeded because she was finally able to discuss her lack of fitness openly. For most participants, the support of others was the greatest factor in their success. Many planned to continue working as a team.

Collectively we had tapped into the power to make changes in our lives. We had set in motion the possibility of realizing our dreams. Working together, we found, made us realize that we didn't have to remain imprisoned. With the support of others, we could shape our bodies—fat or fit—and, along with our bodies, our lives! When we overcame the secret shame of being overweight by telling ourselves and others the truth, and when we joined others to get fit, we took control of own destinies—a heady experience!

Being part of a larger group effort, it turned out, had allowed participants to rediscover a sense of belonging.

Summing It Up: Getting Fit Together

I sorted through the comments, noticing themes. I took note of what people had appreciated and what had worked well for them. Over time, three simple principles emerged. Through intuition more than through conscious planning, I had built these three elements into the Meltdown—and into my individual makeover as well.

And no wonder! The three concepts were embedded in my approach to living. They were the same principles that had informed my teaching, my parenting, and my professional business career. I just was a little slow in applying them to help me tackle fitness.

They were simple and straightforward ideas:

- I love to have fun.

- I believe in the uniqueness of the individual.

- I delight in being part of a team.

It's no surprise, then, that these threads were woven into the fabric of the Meltdown.

F: Fun

We made it *fun* so people would participate.

Whether it was eating, exercising, or meeting in groups, everyone had tons of fun. Some teams met during the week to talk together; some met for a light lunch and friendship. Others sewed matching outfits to wear to meetings. Many teammates shared recipes and exchanged calorie-cutting cooking tips. Almost all called or e-mailed each other when they needed support.

Their team names reflected their attitude: Tons of Fun, We've Got the Spirit, Baby Bimbos, Belly Busters, Better Weight Than Ever, Big Losers, Circle of Friends, Fab-U-Less, Fatanators, Friends for Life, Friendship Club, Great Expectations, Half Ton of Fun, Health Nuts, Just for the Health of It, Soar Losers, Team Wannabeslim, Lettuce Begin, LoCal Locals, Pound Busters, Seven Amigos, Shape Shifters, Shrinking Violets, and Thin to Win, to name a few.

Participants shared a contagious spirit of adventure, along with the joy of learning new skills. They experimented with ways of exercising they had never before considered—from Bikram yoga to bicycling, from fencing to racquetball, from Jazzercise to jumping rope. Classes that offered follow-up sessions on eating or back care were quickly filled. For many, exercise became a form of play rather than a "to do" competing with other tasks. It also began to be incorporated into each day's routine instead of being exceptional. And with so many people engaged in an effort to become fit, everyone and everything around us became our teacher.

I: Individualized/Integrated

Individual needs were met so people could *integrate* changes into their daily lives.

One size does not fit all. Because, to be sustainable, changes had to be integrated into the daily routine of life, each person needed to find healthful ways of eating that they personally enjoyed. Dieting was discouraged because it came from someone else's idea of what works, not from within each person; plus, it was a short-term fix that could not be sustained. Health benefits, such as weight loss and lowered blood pressure, although valuable, were not the goal—they were by-products of day-by-day healthful, individual choices, which, because they were integrated into daily life, became habitual.

Individualism extended to exercise. The choice and purpose of the exercise was up to the individual, but it was essential to be consistent— to integrate it into everyday life. Some participants wanted to improve their balance and flexibility; others wanted to lose weight. Still others exercised to fend off stiffening arthritic joints or reduce medication by lowering their blood pressure. Some individuals liked solo exercise and used the time for meditation and creative thinking; others liked to be surrounded by friends who made the time spent exercising fly. Some needed gentle exercise, such as walking in a pool; others were ready to tackle demanding sports, like tennis. The goal was the same—to become as fit as possible; the means had to be tailored to the individual so that each person could integrate it into his or her daily routine.

T: Together

We made it a team effort, doing it *together*.

We need each other. Most of us can't make significant lifestyle changes— especially losing weight—on our own. Most of us can't find the willpower to exercise regularly by ourselves.

We also need the advice of professionals in health care and related disciplines to move safely toward fitness. Thus during the Meltdown we asked for help from professionals from a variety of disciplines—a physician, physical therapist, dietitian, nurse-practitioner, psychologist, and personal trainer, just to name a few. We also asked for and received institutional and program support from local fitness centers and weight loss centers.

The greatest support, though, came from each other on a day-to-day basis. Building a community of teams—whether they were neighbors, coworkers, fellow congregants, family, or new friends—provided us with a way to give and receive regular feedback and encouragement.

We had *fun*, we made *individual* choices that we could *integrate* into our daily routine, and we achieved results *together*.

) (

Take the Leap:
Seven Steps to Personal Fitness

Either you decide to stay in the shallow end of the pool,
or you go out in the ocean.

CHRISTOPHER REEVE

You've come this far. Give in to your impulse to realize your dream. Do you want to feel better about your body? Do you want to give up some troublesome habits, like overeating at night? Do you want to be a better example for your children? Are you concerned about a spouse? Do you have a medical condition that will cost you your life if you don't adopt healthier habits? Are you concerned about rising health costs and eager to avoid chronic diseases as you age? Whatever reason you have for wanting to change is unique to you. Give in to your heart's desire to have your life match your dream.

You don't have to be special. Be assured that the people I've written about in this book who are working toward their dream are ordinary people. They don't have exceptional willpower or unlimited resources. What they do have is the willingness to take the following seven steps. Take a look at them. Perhaps then you will join us.

Seven Steps to Personal Fitness

1. Fork in the Road, Not in the Mouth

Decide: Your decision to change must be authentic and self-generated. It may be triggered by a medical emergency or by a traumatic incident, such as a stranger asking you if you are pregnant (and you aren't). The decision is inspired from inside you, it is nonreversible, and it will change your life. It is also renewable—when you drift away, a nagging sense that you are off track will bring you back. Your priorities are altered. Wherever you turn, you see validation for the changes you are making. Like the person who learns a new word and sees it everywhere, your commitment to fitness shows up all around you. Timing is everything. If you haven't had this moment of truth, don't despair. Keep looking for the opportunity to step out. You will know it the instant it occurs.

2. Tell the Truth

Go Public: Your decision to get fit once and for all must be communicated as widely as possible. You need to tell your family, and certainly your spouse or significant other. Ask for prayers for your project in your church bulletin, or announce your goal at synagogue. You can make your resolve known in your social or service clubs or post it on the bulletin board at work. You can even take an ad out in a newspaper. Have fun! Trust me, you will find all sorts of people who will support your efforts, and some may even join you in getting fit.

3. Find "My People"

Assemble a Team: I recently heard a psychiatrist talk about the importance of separating the people you come in contact with into two groups: "my people" and "not my people." She said it makes life much more enjoyable if you surround yourself with "my people" and give up guilt about dissociating yourself from the others. It is easy to recognize "not my people." They make you feel bad when you are around them; you shrink before their critical gaze. Their unhappiness is toxic. Stick with "my people," who give you a lift and make you happy to be alive.

Now that you have gone public and announced your decision to make a life change, the next step is to assemble a team for personal and professional support—a team of "my people." The professional members might include a personal trainer, physician, physical therapist, psychologist, acupuncturist, and/or dietitian. Consider a hospital wellness center that offers a health and risk assessment.

Work with your doctor, and get medical tests to find out if you have any issues or limitations that need to be addressed. Personal support might involve a Weight Watchers group, Take Off Pounds Sensibly (TOPS), classmates in a gym group, friends who want to join you in getting fit, your spouse, or neighbors. Remember—overweight or out-of-shape people are not scarce. You can create your support team from almost any group in which you participate.

4. From Fat to Fit

Set Goals and Design Your Own Program: Once you have your team, you need to design your own unique fitness program. You must set goals and then decide how you will reach them. Here are some examples:

Weight Loss:

- I will lose thirty pounds in six months.
- My eating plan will include foods that I find enjoyable (within limits!) but with a focus on health and nutrition. This means a lot of fresh fruits and vegetables.
- I'll eat breakfast daily and will record faithfully all that I consume.
- My diet will include a maximum of 1,500 calories a day.
- I'll learn the calorie content of food and how to read labels.

Exercise:

- Unless I'm injured or sick, I will exercise an average of one hour a day, or a total of seven hours each week.
- I will find exercises that improve my flexibility, build strength through resistance training (weights), and engage in aerobic activities that provide overall conditioning.
- I will explore and find exercise that is intrinsically fun and rewarding.

Project Management:

- I will establish the number of inches I want to lose and measure myself at the start so that I have a benchmark.

- Each week I'll take new measurements and record the changes. When pounds don't drop as easily or as much as I want, I'll take encouragement from my declining inches.

- Each week I will report my results to my fitness coach and will set new goals.

- I will make a list of healthy habits that I regularly need to observe to take good care of myself. My first items are staying hydrated, flossing my teeth daily, wearing a seat belt, getting sufficient sleep, and balancing my commitments between work, family, and self.

- Regarding my mental health, I'll find an opportunity to laugh each day, give attention to my spiritual needs, and maintain a fun, upbeat outlook.

- When people notice changes in me, I'll use the opportunity to encourage them to join me in choosing a healthier lifestyle.

5. In the Card Game of Life, Honesty Trumps Denial

Establish Accountability: Two kinds of accountability are necessary. Self-accountability means daily journaling of what you eat, how much you exercise, and what your attitude is. For this you need your own personal journal. One way is to manually log in daily information in a notebook that you have created. An alternative is to set up your reporting system on your computer. Or you can use a free Web-based program like the one you can find at http://www.fitday.com. For a small fee, you can also use a popular commercial site: http://www.myfooddiary.com.

Keep handy a pen or pencil and something to write on, like a pad of paper, next to your favorite chair. Or buy a small notebook that you can fit into your purse or pocket. This makes it easy to journal wherever you are.

You also need to report weekly to an outside source. This could be a team member, a supporter, or a personal trainer. Left to our own devices, we tend to deny unpleasant realities. Consequently, this last step is absolutely essential to reach your goals.

6. Become a Student Again

Learn, Experiment, and Celebrate: Be prepared for a major learning curve in all areas of your life. You will need to learn new ways of cooking and dining out. Make notes of how different foods affect your body. Make a ritual of eating, paying special attention to portion size. (For fifty-six tips on cooking and eating, see appendix A.) Experiment with different forms of exercise. Celebrate progress. As you lose weight, make adjustments in your wardrobe by donating clothes that are too big. (I found consignment stores great places to find an interim wardrobe while I was going down in sizes.)

Continue to research fitness through a variety of sources—books, magazines, Web sites, your physician and pharmacist, and your local fitness center. (See appendix B for Web site sources.) Learn to accept and enjoy change, variety, experimentation, and the joy of celebration. The journey of learning, growing, changing, and adapting is one that will last for the rest of your life.

7. Recruit or Regress

Promote and Institutionalize: "Sell" fitness to your family members and business associates and to members of groups you belong to. Become the self-appointed fitness advocate in your circle of friends and neighbors

The Plan of Action

- The plan of action must be written. In this process, you are reprogramming yourself to behave differently.

- Actions must be specific and located in time—for example, each week, each day. Vagueness and ambiguity don't serve us.

- Actions must be measurable. That is, you can easily determine whether you followed through and whether progress is being made. We need encouragement during the journey. Measuring our progress is a big boost.

- Actions must be monitored for compliance by someone other than yourself. At first, we can't be our own monitor; we need the help of others. That leads us to our next action.

and in the larger community. Find a group of people who will reinforce your new lifestyle, and make them your new friends. To institutionalize your own changes at home, keep only one size of clothing in your closet. Show guests the kitchen cupboard along with the refrigerator. Their contents reflect your new way of eating. Use every opportunity you can to encourage others to join you in leading a more healthful life.

One Last Word of Encouragement

Don't feel you have to accomplish each of these seven steps perfectly. None of us moves flawlessly toward our goals. We take spills and detours along the way. Besides, there is no destination, only the journey. All we have are day-to-day, moment-by-moment decisions to make.

And you don't have to wait for the perfect opportunity or the perfect words to encourage others. Instead, share yourself and your enthusiasm for your new lifestyle in your own unique way.

You may be surprised that as you begin to reinvent the new "you," latent interests and talents begin to surface. Once you permit yourself freedom in one area of your life, that freedom becomes available to you in other areas as well. In ways you least expect it, your newfound freedom will begin to transform the rest of your life. Fortunately, we don't need to understand how it works to appreciate the wonderful outcome when we begin to make healthful changes in support of our bodies.

Dying with Our Potential Intact—the Ultimate Tragedy

When I look back on my decision to get fit, I am frightened. What if, I ask myself, I had not changed my ways? Most likely, I would not be alive, and I certainly wouldn't be writing this book. It seems to me that the greatest crime is to die with our potential intact; the greatest joy is to spill that potential into the world and become the person we were intended to be.

You too can realize your heart's desire!

And in doing so, you will help others do the same.

Run with the Big Dogs!
Seven Steps to Community Fitness

You can run with the big dogs
or sit on the porch and bark.

WALLACE ARNOLD

Once you are reasonably confident that you have achieved stability in your own new lifestyle, your next task is to step out and lead others. By putting yourself in a leadership position in your community, as I accidentally did with the Meltdown, you reinforce your own commitment to live healthfully while giving to others.

Does it frighten you to think about stepping out? Does it scare you to contemplate creating an event in your own community? Maybe it will help if you think of the experience as exhilarating—because that is what it will be if you dare attempt it.

"Now" probably doesn't seem like a good time either, does it? Are you thinking that maybe some point in time in the future would be better? Yet "now" is all we have. Yesterday is gone and tomorrow may never happen. And when tomorrow does arrive, it will probably have the same limitations you are facing now. There is never a perfect time; the only perfect time is now.

Bloom Where You're Planted

My advice: use any season of your life to begin. If it is the start of the new year, offer a program that features fresh aspirations. If it's spring, let the new growth around you tap the impulse for a new beginning. If it's summer, use those long days to organize outdoor exercise meetings.

Fall, on the other hand, is a time for school and learning. So buy a school notebook and use its fresh, blank sheets to organize a community event. If you're headed into the holidays, give your neighbors and friends a boost with a program to nourish their spirits instead of filling their plates. Whatever the time, go for it!

Use whatever community you are in: if you're working full time, organize your fellow employees. If you're a stay-at-home parent, organize your neighbors and friends. If you're retired, organize the seniors around you. If you're a member of a church, begin with your fellow congregants. Maybe you can organize a program for family members using e-mail. Or maybe you live in a high-rise apartment and can get like-minded residents to participate in a program. Wherever you are, you can find others who need the changes you've been making in your own life. Who better than you to invite them to participate?

And don't feel constrained by the structure of our Meltdown. Feel free to create your own unique event, or hook up with like-minded people to create a wholly different kind of fitness project. Feel free to innovate and create the program that is uniquely right for you and your community.

Stepping Out Together: Can We Create an Epidemic of Fitness?

If enough of us step out, we can trigger a fitness epidemic. Despite the grim statistics in the newspaper, many of us are making positive changes in an attempt to achieve a more healthful lifestyle. What most convinces me are changes occurring with my immediate family and circle of friends. Dick is taking an exercise class three times a week and playing tennis twice a week, and he is careful about what he eats. Steve, my son who lives in France, has trimmed down and exercises regularly. Marc, my second child, is increasingly concerned about his fitness—a precursor to making changes. Granddaughters—who never met a hamburger and french fry they didn't love—now join me for Subway sandwiches. Dinner guests appreciate low-calorie fare.

Retailers are getting into the act. Grocery stores have added health-conscious food products and choices that didn't exist months ago. Food networks feature "cooking thin" shows. Newspapers and magazines—from *Guideposts* to *Business Week*—regularly feature articles on fitness. Applebee's introduced eight Weight Watchers appetizers, entrées, and desserts. Other chains have jumped on the bandwagon, offering salads and low-carb options.

At what point are there enough fitness fanatics to reach the tipping point? The point where the trend toward obesity is reversed? The point where we replace an epidemic of obesity with an epidemic of fitness?

Shift Happens

Twenty years ago cigarette smoking was common everywhere and among all classes of people. Nonsmokers were in the minority. Secondhand smoke was accepted in restaurants, public buildings, and even in the enclosed space of an airline. Smoking was glamorized in movies.

Over time the adverse impact on our health became indisputable. Public opinion changed; smoking was no longer a desirable, sophisticated habit. Rather it was an addiction that took a toll on the health and pocketbook of the smoker.

Of course, not everyone has stopped smoking. But the shift in public attitude has resulted in a wide range of changes throughout our society. Smoke-free restaurants, hotels, and car rentals are now routinely available. Smoking on airplanes is forbidden. Parents and school administrators discourage their teenagers from taking up the habit. A huge shift has occurred in a relatively short amount of time.

The same shift needs to occur to help us return to a more normal weight and regular exercise.

How will this shift take place? All it takes is a few committed individuals, like you and me. We will be scattered throughout communities across the nation. First we will take personal responsibility for making healthful lifestyle choices for ourselves. Then we will step off the porch and begin to work together with our neighbors and friends to make changes in our schools, at work, and in our homes.

Seven Steps Toward Community Fitness

For those of you who are ready to step off the porch and lead your own community fitness project, here is your list of actions. Use this list so you can make sure your plans are complete. And remember—although your program may focus on fitness and losing tons of fat, the most wonderful by-product will be the revitalized sense of the power of community to improve our lives.

1. Catalytic Converter

Turn Ideas into Action: One person, a catalyst, must decide to create a community fitness event and then seek support from others to create a core group that will make it happen. If you aren't the catalyst, then find one or join like-minded groups. You will know this person or the appropriate group by their eagerness to take a leadership role.

2. Create Magic and Power

Go Public: Choose a clever name that has broad appeal and impact. Announce the plan and the goal—to help friends and neighbors lose weight and get fit. If you are going to do a communitywide event, consider including churches, synagogues, mosques, radio and television stations, newspapers, gyms, government offices, hospitals, private medical practices, and schools.

3. Use the Synergy of Teamwork

Assemble Support: Assemble a team of ten to twelve people who represent a cross section of your community. For example, select leaders from the medical community, private businesses, government offices, and educational organizations. Find those who share your passion about fitness. This becomes the nucleus group, where decisions can be quickly made and implemented.

4. Eyes to See and Hands to Do

Set Goals and Create Structure: Articulate your vision, pick a start date, determine measurements for success, and promote via all available venues (television, radio, newspapers, e-mail networks, and so forth). Ask for volunteer help. Tap in to existing volunteer or fitness groups willing to make a contribution to the larger effort. For example, talk to a local running club or hiking club. They will have members who want to promote fitness. This will involve recruiting and assigning point people to key jobs—public relations, recruitment and supervision of volunteers, facility management, business and insurance, event production, program presentations, public relations and promotion, communications, and operations.

Establish policies, and announce the names of the point people who have authority to make decisions on behalf of the project. Design your kickoff program to include format, subjects for presentation, and length. Invite well-known speakers to make presentations at events; publicize their appearances in advance. Be sure to plan your concluding program around a theme of celebration.

5. Each Other's Keeper

Establish a System of Accountability: Create a way for participants to team together. Establish a captain for each team. Help each team establish its baseline, set goals, and set up an internal communication system. For the larger group, establish an e-mail–based communication system, which can be used for reporting individual, team, and group results to a central party who can collect and distribute the results. This party can also use e-mail to communicate announcements, form new teams, and announce prizes.

Publicly acknowledging victories has a synergistic effect. To bring the community effort into the public arena, create a dedicated Web site and feedback loop via local television stations, newspapers, and radio stations. Create a community blog where individuals and teams can share stories, exchange recipes and clothes, challenge other teams, ask about resources, find a team to join, or line up rides to meetings.

6. Students in the University of Life

Learn, Experiment, and Celebrate: After each event, meet and critique. Based on these insights plus other program needs, consider including the following elements:

- Celebrate weekly successes.

- Establish weekly goals.

- Dramatize progress in meaningful ways during the events.

- Publicize positive results through media.

- Encourage team members to attend fitness events dressed alike with clothes themed around their team name.

7. Make the Time, Make the Commitment, to Actively Advocate

Encourage Activism on Behalf of Health and Well-Being: Encourage participants to "sell" fitness. Arrange to have buttons and T-shirts for participants to wear during and after the event. Empower participants to become self-appointed fitness advocates in their own circle of friends, among their neighbors, and in the larger community. Encourage them to contact their elected officials, write to their local newspaper, and make their voices heard in any available forum.

Convert idealism to action. Work to bring positive change in schools (healthier food choices for students), in restaurants (posting caloric content of food and healthier choices), and in your local newspaper (add or expand the fitness page). Sponsor and support events in the community of like-minded people. Find and associate with persons interested in promoting fitness in the community. Before long, you'll have a powerful network of people with whom you can work to bring about community change.

From Fat to Fit Together

Whether you work on your own personal makeover or lead a community effort, I encourage you to undertake your tasks in a spirit of fun, adventure, and learning. Experimenting with our own bodies and our own communities, we can make new choices leading to healthier lifestyles. Just as we had fun getting fat together, we can have fun getting fit together. The difference is the outcome—one produces guilt and depression, the other freedom and joy!

) (

What Have You Got to Lose?
What Have You Got to Gain?

You miss 100 percent of the shots you never take.
WAYNE GRETZKY

With a sense of urgency, I'm doing what I can to promote fitness, first by shaping up myself, and then by persuading people in my community to join me. Beyond that, I've written this book to convey to you how much fun and joy we shared along the way. My hope is that our enthusiasm is contagious—that it will take up residence in your heart and you will be unable to resist joining the effort.

Because, truly, the next step is yours. Are you committed to living healthfully? Would you like to roll back the clock on aging and enjoy a new vitality and zest for living? Are you willing to change today's routine so you can enjoy a thousand healthy tomorrows?

Are you willing to go beyond yourself and serve as an example for your family, friends, and fellow travelers through life? Are you willing to be a catalyst to promote fitness in your community? If so, may you step forward and, without knowing the full implications of your commitment, say publicly: "Count me in!"

Only you can decide your next course of action. You can put this book down and go on with your life as before. Or you can grab hold of our vision and bring it to your community.

You needn't have the resources at your fingertips to begin. I didn't. All you need is a resolve to step forward and claim fitness for yourself and your family, your friends and neighbors, and your community. All you need to do is begin.

Trust me, the resources will flow to you at exactly the moment you need them. Fitness is an idea whose time has come. More and more of us are becoming weapons of mass reduction. Through the testimony of how we live our lives, we make a contribution to the larger effort.

Step out. Step forward.

Welcome to the future!

Appendices

Fifty-six Discoveries about Eating and Cooking

Here are fifty-six discoveries I've made while working on my own fitness. I continue to update the list as I learn more about my body and how it reacts to food and exercise. As you pursue your fitness goals, I suggest you create your own list. Test these discoveries against your own experience to see which ones work for you. Learning and experimenting are fun!

1. **Timing:** Eat at periodic intervals (about four hours). Don't skip a meal or wait until you are starved. Otherwise you will overeat or make poor eating choices. Have a snack planned (fruit is good) to eat after you take a daytime rest/nap; otherwise, you will crave something with sugar (for example, piece of cake or candy bar) and won't be able to resist. If you do have a sweet treat, deduct it from your daily calorie allowance.

2. **Breakfast:** Always eat breakfast. Include protein (egg whites scrambled), carbohydrate (whole wheat toast with no-fat spray butter), dairy (nonfat cottage cheese), and fruit (for example, a grapefruit).

3. **Volume:** In the colder seasons, make a big pot of vegetable soup at the start of the week to have on hand for quick lunches or for filling up before dinner. Use cabbage and eggplant as main vegetables. Add celery, carrots, onions, leeks, mushrooms, and chopped canned

tomatoes. Use chicken broth and/or bouillon for flavoring. Leave out potatoes and pasta. In the warmer seasons, make big salads and keep a bowl of cut-up fruit.

4. **Snacks:** Have a snack about 4:00 PM (popcorn, either air popped or low-cal microwave) and add fruit if you are especially hungry. Add some hot herbal tea. It's more difficult to overeat if your stomach is already nearly full. Fruit also helps take away a sugar craving.

5. **Protein:** To keep energy up, make sure you have protein in every meal. Low-calorie sources of protein include fat-free cottage cheese, soy, fish, poached white meat of chicken, and tuna.

6. **Managing Hunger:** Have a piece or two of rye bread when you are especially hungry and can't wait for mealtime.

7. **More on Hunger:** Treat hunger as your best friend. That is, when you get hungry, you know you are burning off fat calories. If you are never hungry, chances are you are gaining weight. You normally will wake up hungry unless you overate the night before.

8. **No Skipping Meals:** Even if you overate the night before and the scale is up, don't skip breakfast. It starts your engine for the day. Don't skip lunch either; you'll be tempted to overeat at night. Balance your calories throughout the day. Don't eat 80 percent of your calories after 5:00 PM.

9. **Replacing Shortening:** Use puréed fresh fruit (such as strawberries), applesauce, or nonfat yogurt in place of oil or shortening for cake mixes, brownies, bread, etc. (I keep the little half-cups of applesauce in the cupboard for this purpose.) The applesauce or yogurt keeps the baked goods moist and enriches flavor. Add decaf coffee concentrate to chocolate desserts to deepen flavor without adding calories.

10. **Special Occasions:** Give yourself a break on holidays and special occasions and eat what you want. Allow yourself to eat along with your guests as long as this isn't more than once every couple of weeks.

11. **Weighing Routine:** Weigh yourself only once a day, at the same time, naked, preferably at the start of the day. Or do it once a week, but be consistent in how you do it.

12. **Alcohol:** Save alcohol (beer, wine, cocktails) for special occasions.

13. **Poaching:** Poach fish in bouillon (fish) and lemon juice.

14. **Spray Oil:** Use spray on products instead of oil when "frying." Use Enova if you need to fry.

15. **Appetite Management:** Always have one dish at each meal that you can eat as much as you want of in case you feel the need for seconds. (My favorite is baked zucchini in chopped tomatoes with onions and seasoned with herbes de Provence.)

16. **Close the Kitchen:** Clean the kitchen after dinner and close it down so you won't be tempted to eat any more.

17. **Sampling Food:** Resist the impulse to sample food when cooking or the impulse to have samples when putting food away, for example, one last bite.

18. **Hungry Days:** If you are having a "hungry" day, double up on vegetables: carrots, zucchini, salad, tomatoes, cucumbers, eggplant, etc.

19. **Water:** Drink lots of water each day.

20. **Fruits for Snacks:** Use fruits for snacks and to manage hunger. Grapes are good. An apple takes a while to eat. Grapefruit makes a nice dessert. You can bake an apple with a little cinnamon and vanilla for a special dessert.

21. **Quick Protein:** Keep a couple of hard-boiled eggs in the refrigerator for a quick protein fix.

22. **Keep Rested:** You make better decisions about what to eat, cook, etc., when rested. Get sufficient sleep at night so that the appetite-regulating hormones can do their job. Sometimes just being tired can trigger a huge appetite.

23. **Leftovers:** If you cook in quantity, freeze or give away anything but the most immediate portions.

24. **Sugar:** In recipes calling for sugar, either use a substitute (Splenda) or reduce the amount of sugar. In many recipes, you can cut the sugar in half without compromising the taste.

25. **Add First Courses:** Start meals with a bowl of soup, preferably a lower calorie one like broth. In summer, begin with chilled soups. The volume reduces the need for large portions for the remainder of the meal.

26. **Manage Kitchen Inventory:** Look through your cupboard and refrigerator. Can you eat what's there and be healthy? If you can't, get rid of it and don't bring it into the house. My downfall—Oreo cookies. I don't dare bring them home because I will eat every last one of them. If you make desserts for the family, put the desserts in an inaccessible and not immediately visible place in the refrigerator. This strategy will help everyone eat less dessert.

27. **Use Distraction:** If you have an hour before you eat and you're hungry, distract yourself with some task that requires all of your attention, like sewing or reading. If that doesn't work, have a cup of hot tea.

28. **Change Your Wardrobe:** Once you've lost weight, get rid of your clothes or tailor them to your new size. That way, if you start gaining weight, you have nothing to wear, the increased size will be noticeable to you, and you can't go into denial about it.

29. **Record:** Keep a record of what you eat so you won't be the King or Queen of Denial. Buy or create your own good calorie counting chart; keep it handy in the kitchen. When you finish cleaning the kitchen, make your final entries for the day, along with the hours of exercise.

30. **Variety:** Vary the content of meals but keep the pattern the same: fruit, protein, vegetables, low-cal dairy, and low-cal bread (such as sourdough).

31. **Limit Meat:** Use meat in small quantities to add flavor to your dish but make a main dish out of vegetables—for example, a stuffed bell pepper with a little bit of ground beef in the filling.

32. **Portion Size:** Pay attention to portion size at every meal. Don't allow yourself second portions. Don't eat more because you exercised that day; otherwise, you are defeating the purpose of exercising.

33. **See Food–Eat Food—How to Manage:** It's easy when you see others indulging, especially in restaurants or fast food places, to feel sorry for yourself. Banish that emotion and instead smugly congratulate yourself on how good you are being. If you must eat fast food, look for salad bars or veggie burgers.

34. **Fall Down and Get Back Up:** If you fall off track, get right back on track at the next meal. Don't overcompensate by starving yourself. This only creates its own set of problems.

35. **Recovering from Alcohol:** If you drink alcohol, be prepared to have sugar cravings the following day. Have a plan ready to deal with sugar cravings (for example, extra fruit or extra activity, preferably away from the house).

36. **Avoid Caffeine:** Except in tea, stay away from caffeine. It stimulates appetite and makes you anxious—both can lead to overeating.

37. **Read Labels:** Read the labels on the backs of products to see what's in them—calories, fat, and chemicals—so you know what you are eating.

38. **Pressure from Others:** If others pressure you to join them in over-indulging, you need to examine the basis of the friendship. You can excuse yourself by saying you ate earlier or you are going to be eating later and don't want to spoil your appetite.

39. **Seamless Dining:** When a guest, don't make a big deal about your special dietary needs. Find something that the host/hostess serves that you can eat and focus on that.

40. **Salad Dressings:** Use lemon juice and rice vinegar on fresh salad in lieu of oil/vinegar.

41. **Find Other Sources of Pleasure:** Give yourself other treats (for example, massage, walk outdoors, phone call to a friend) to replace the comforts you were getting from food.

42. **Self-Medicating:** If you need medicine, take it. Don't self-medicate with food or alcohol.

43. **Go Nutty:** Eat some nuts occasionally. A small/tiny handful will give you enough fat to make you feel satisfied.

44. **Use Buttermilk:** Add dissolved unflavored gelatin to buttermilk to make no-fat sour cream unless you want to buy the commercial version.

45. **Plan Ahead:** Create menus and dishes you will look forward to eating. Focus on what you can eat—not what you can't have or what you are depriving yourself of. Eat foods you like that are good for you.

46. **Enjoy Eating:** Food is life, according to the French, and eating should be a pleasurable experience. Set the table and arrange food on the plates for visual appeal. Use spices to create variety and to satisfy the need for different kinds of tastes. Turn off the TV; don't read. Give your full attention to the pleasurable enjoyment of nourishing your body.

47. **Entertaining:** When you entertain, serve foods that will be a treat to guests but always serve something that you can eat as well. If, for example, you have nuts and cheese to serve with cocktails, then make sure you also have low-fat popcorn. If you have a rich, calorie-dense dinner, make sure there are vegetables and salad you can eat.

48. **Fast Food on the Road:** Eat Subway sandwiches for lunches when traveling on the road. Subway restaurants are everywhere, and the turkey sandwich on whole wheat without cheese or mayo is only 300 calories. Add some hot tea and you will feel very full.

49. **Chew Gum:** If you're hungry and it isn't time to eat yet, chew a stick of no-calorie gum. It satisfies the urge to chew without adding any calories.

50. **Grocery Shopping:** Shop for groceries when you are not overly hungry. Stick to your shopping list.

51. **Learn and Experiment:** Try new recipes. Try new foods. Try different ways of fixing family favorites so that they contain fewer calories. Buy some cookbooks that feature nourishing but lower calorie menus. Buy some new kitchen toys to use with your experiments.

52. **Eating Out:** Decide before you go into a restaurant what you are going to eat. Don't be afraid to ask for special preparation. Keep bread and butter out of your immediate reach. Take half or more of your dinner home if portions are large. Split your entrée with your partner if she or he is being conscious of calories. If someone at the table orders dessert, sample it and enjoy the sample. But stop there.

53. **Whole Wheat Grains:** Switch over to whole wheat bread, pasta, and flour. The whole wheat pastry flour is light enough to use in baking and gives a nutty flavor. Besides providing nutrients, whole grain is more filling and helps you manage your appetite.

54. **Cheese:** Use cheese sparingly. Stick with the hard cheeses, such as Parmesan, which are less calorie dense but still add flavor. Use cheddar and other softer cheeses for flavoring. Usually you can cut down the amount of cheese a recipe calls for by half and still have sufficient cheese flavor. If a casserole recipe includes cheese, then eliminate meat from the menu and make the pasta/cheese dish the entrée.

55. **Enjoy Food Preparation:** Many of the lower calorie dishes involve physical acts, such as chopping, slicing, and mixing. Cooking also challenges us to be creative and playful. After you sit down to eat, take the time to enjoy not only the meal but also the gift that meal preparation represents. Preparing and serving wonderful, nutritious, and healthy food is a way of saying "I care."

56. **To Shrink the Belly, Shrink the Plate:** Serve your meals on salad plates instead of full-size dinner plates. Your plate will seem fuller, so you'll feel as if you have a sufficient quantity to eat. Using a smaller plate will also help you choose and eat the appropriate portion size for your meals.

Web Site Resources

The Internet can be a wonderful source of information about weight loss, fitness, and health issues—if you know where to look. This section lists Web sites that we have found to be useful sources of reliable information. The listings highlight the best features of each site, but if you keep browsing you'll also find useful articles, links to other interesting sites, free e-mail newsletters, blogs, and much more.

Children

Childhood obesity and children's nutrition are important issues for families and communities. These sites offer information you'll find useful for your own children or grandchildren or the children in your community.

Center for Science in the Public Interest
http://www.cspinet.org/nutritionpolicy/index.html

Find out how food companies market to children by reading the eye-opening report, "Pestering Parents: How Food Companies Market Obesity to Children." Follow up with "Guidelines for Responsible Food Marketing to Children," developed to help companies manufacture, sell, market, and promote food to children in a manner that encourages healthy eating.

GirlsHealth.gov
http://www.girlshealth.gov/

Reliable information for girls (ages ten to sixteen) about fitness, nutrition, health issues, and other topics from the National Women's Health

Information Center, part of the U.S. Department of Health and Human Services.

MedlinePlus
http://www.nlm.nih.gov/medlineplus/exerciseforchildren.html
Find links to news and articles about exercise for children from the U.S. National Library of Medicine and the National Institutes of Health. Available in Spanish.

The National Alliance for Nutrition and Activity
http://www.schoolwellnesspolicies.org
Model School Wellness Policies
This set of policies for physical activity and nutrition was developed to help local school districts write and implement wellness policies consistent with the Child Nutrition and WIC Reauthorization Act of 2004. Sixty health, nutrition, physical activity, and education organizations worked together to create these model school wellness policies.

Diet and Nutrition

At these sites, you'll find an abundance of useful information about eating, presented in an entertaining and colorful way.

American Dietetic Association
http://www.eatright.org
Nutritional information from the nation's largest organization of food and nutrition professionals.

American Heart Association
http://www.americanheart.org
Advice about what's good to eat and what isn't.

American Institute for Cancer Research
http://www.aicr.org/hotline
Dietitians will provide free answers by phone or e-mail to nutrition questions within three days. While you're waiting, browse through answers to popular queries or check out the Recipe Corner. (800) 843-8114.

Diet.com
http://www.diet.com
Take the Diet Personality Test and learn how your personality influences dieting success.

The Diet Detective
http://www.Nutricise.com

Find articles, tips, community forums, interviews with leading health experts, and a free newsletter from Charles Stuart Platkin, author of the "Diet Detective" column.

eDiets.com
http://www.eDiets.com

If you're a private person or someone who is too busy to go to a weekly meeting, support online has never been easier to find or use. This site offers support groups, a mentor program, and a chat room, plus articles, tips, and a free e-mail newsletter.

Portion Distortion
http://hp2010.nhlbihin.net/portion/

Quizzes from the National Heart, Lung, and Blood Institute test your knowledge of how portion size has changed over the years. For example, a bagel in 1984 was three inches wide and had 140 calories; today it's six inches and 350 calories. You'll also find a handy wallet-size card to remind you what a standard food serving looks like.

Time Magazine Food Quiz
http://www.time.com/time/covers/20060612/quiz/

Test how much you know about the food you eat.

U.S. Department of Agriculture
http://www.ars.usda.gov/ba/bhnrc/ndl

Find free calorie counts for most foods.

WebMD
http://www.webmd.com

This popular site offers weight control, weight loss, and nutritional guidance in the Healthy Living section.

Exercise

These sites will educate you about exercise of all types and help keep you motivated.

About.com
http://www.walking.about.com/

This popular site offers a comprehensive section on walking as an accessible, inexpensive way to achieve ongoing fitness. Explore topics such as common mistakes new walkers make, wearing the right shoes, walking clubs, and much more.

American Council on Exercise
http://www.acefitness.org

Find fitness tips, recipes, and information on how to become a fitness trainer.

America on the Move Foundation
http://www.Americaonthemove.org

This organization provides free Web-based programs, tools, and resources to individuals, families, groups, and communities of all types and sizes, including a customized goal-setting feature and log to track your progress.

American Volkssport Association
http://www.ava.org

You can search by state to find a list of walking clubs or events in your area or in places you may be visiting. Most walks are free.

The Aquatic Exercise Association
http://www.aeawave.com

This not-for-profit association offers information about the benefits of aquatic exercise.

"Exercise: The Key to the Good Life"
http://www.fitness.gov/pepup.htm
Also available in pdf: http://www.fitness.gov/pepup.pdf

This booklet from the President's Council on Physical Fitness and Sports offers a program of simple exercises to improve flexibility, strength, and endurance. Many can be done from a chair or wheelchair.

Map My Run
http://www.mapmyrun.com/

Instead of a pedometer, try this high-tech approach to your fitness routine. Plot your run or walk on this site and then calculate how far you walked, your speed, calories burned, and more.

Measure My Effort
http://www.gmap-pedometer.com

Whether you're jogging, walking, or biking, measure your effort with the Gmaps Pedometer. Enter the address where you start your route, and zoom in or out until you see your path. Then hit the "start recording" button and mark your route to find out the total distance. You can also see calories burned and difficulty and journal your accomplishments.

MedlinePlus
http://www.nlm.nih.gov/medlineplus/exerciseandphysicalfitness.html

News and information about health and fitness from the U.S. National Library of Medicine and the National Institutes of Health. Available in Spanish.

Prevention.com
http://www.prevention.com

Click on Fitness to find lots of information about different types of exercise, especially walking. Find walking tips, quizzes, and how-tos, even podcasts about walking.

Health and Medicine

Whether you need information about drugs, dietary supplements, diseases and treatments, or general health issues, these sites are a great place to start.

Consumer Reports Medical Guide
http://www.consumerreports.org/mg/home.htm

Read free drug reviews, treatment ratings, natural medicine ratings, plus news and safety alerts. Subscribers to the site (by the month or by the year) can access even more information.

Familydoctor.org
http://familydoctor.org

Information about living a healthy lifestyle—with sections for men, women, seniors, and children—from the American Academy of Family Physicians.

HealthierUS.gov
http://www.healthierus.gov

This site offers "credible, accurate information to help Americans choose to live healthier lives." Topics include physical fitness, prevention, nutrition, and making healthy choices.

Mayo Clinic
http://www.mayoclinic.com

Find quizzes, health calculators, and an "ask the expert" section, plus plenty of information about living well or managing a health condition.

Medline
http://www.medlineplus.gov

Find information from the National Library of Medicine on more than seven hundred health topics plus interactive tutorials, links to clinical trials, and the latest health news.

MedWatch
http://www.fda.gov/medwatch

This site from the U.S. Food and Drug Administration provides timely safety information on drugs and other medical products, including the adverse effects of supplements.

The National Association of Anorexia Nervosa and Associated Disorders
http://www.anad.org

This site offers free information and resources for disorders including anorexia, bulimia, and compulsive eating. The organization has over 350 support groups and will help you find one in your area.

National Center for Complementary and Alternative Medicine
http://nccam.nih.gov

This site offers information about complementary and alternative medicine from a respected source, the National Institutes of Health. If you're browsing for health information on the Internet, don't miss the article, "10 Things to Know about Evaluating Medical Resources on the Web."

PatientINFORM
http://www.patientinform.org

This free online service provides patients and their caregivers with access to some of the most up-to-date and reliable research available about the diagnosis and treatment of specific diseases, including cancer, heart disease, and diabetes.

Reader's Digest
http://www.rd.com

Click on Health to find an impressive collection of articles from respected authorities on health and wellness issues, ranging from acupuncture to cosmetic safety. Recipes, health tools, expert advice, and several free e-mail newsletters make this site an invaluable source of information about healthy living.

SupplementWatch.com
http://www.supplementwatch.com

This independent Web site seeks to provide timely, relevant, balanced advice to help consumers make informed decisions about dietary supplements. Professionals analyze the quality and potency of vitamins, minerals, and supplements. Much of the information on the site is free.

University of Maryland Medical Center, Complementary Medicine Program
http://www.umm.edu/altmed

Reputable research on herbal medicine and alternative treatments, including herbs, supplements, and treatment options.

Your Disease Risk
http://www.yourdiseaserisk.harvard.edu/

Complete this free questionnaire from the Harvard Center for Cancer Prevention to find out your risk of developing five of the most important diseases in the United States: cancer, diabetes, heart disease, osteoporosis, and stroke. Then get personalized tips for preventing them.

Integrative Healthcare

Integrative healthcare uses both conventional and complementary techniques and treatments to help patients experience optimal vitality and wellness, no matter what their current state of health. For people seeking integrated care or medical professionals interested in learning more, here are the leading institutions in the nation.

Carolinas Integrative Health, Charlotte, North Carolina
http://www.carolinashealthcare.org/services/CIH/welcome.cfm

Continuum Health Partners, New York City, New York
http://www.wehealnewyork.org

Duke Center for Integrative Medicine, Durham, North Carolina
http://www.dukehealth.org/Services/IntegrativeMedicine/index

Evanston Northwestern Healthcare, Glenview, Illinois
http://www.enh.org/healthandwellness/clinicalservices/integrative/

Maine Medical Center Family Practice Center, Falmouth, Maine
http://www.mmc.org/mmc_body.cfm?id=1990

University of Arizona Program in Integrative Medicine, Tucson, Arizona
http://integrativemedicine.arizona.edu/

University of Wisconsin Center for Integrative Medicine, Madison, Wisconsin
http://www.uwhealth.org

Seniors

Seniors will find help with their special health and fitness needs at these sites.

AARP
http://www.aarp.org/health/fitness/walking/

Information and advice on how to start walking. Order the free Physical Activities Workbook online or call (888) OUR-AARP and ask for stock number D561.

Fifty-Plus Lifelong Fitness
http://www.50plus.org

Find listings of fitness events and information specific to midlife and older adults.

MedlinePlus
http://www.nlm.nih.gov/medlineplus/exerciseforseniors.html

Find links to news and articles about exercise for seniors from the U.S. National Library of Medicine and the National Institutes of Health. Available in Spanish.

NIH Senior Health
http://nihseniorhealth.gov

This site from the National Institutes of Health gives senior-specific health and fitness information, including the option of enlarging text or having text read aloud.

National Institute on Aging
http://www.nia.nih.gov/

Health and research information from the National Institutes of Health. Browse, search, and order publications and other materials. Most are free.

Red Hat Society
http://www.redhatsociety.com

This site offers ways for women to establish social networks, thereby enhancing emotional fitness. Opportunities for play and friendship are organized through local chapters. A walking/exercise program sponsored by AARP promotes fitness.

Senior Journal.com
http://www.seniorjournal.com

Browse fitness news and information for seniors.

Staying Organized

Don't let "paperwork" keep you from your workout. Let these sites do the math and recordkeeping for you.

Calories Per Hour.com
http://www.caloriesperhour.com/index_burn.html

Keep track of calories so you can systematically lose weight and keep it off. Choose from hundreds of activities from accordion playing to yoga.

Cyberdiet
http://www.cyberdiet.com

Log your calories, track your progress, and learn calorie and nutrition information from over forty popular fast food outlets.

DietWatch.com
http://www.dietwatch.com

Although most of the services here are available only to members, the handy nutrition calculator is free. Find calories, vitamins, and other nutritional information about a huge number of foods, often with brand names. (A search for "apple" produced two hundred results—from infant cereal with applesauce to apple-cinnamon tea.)

Family Health Portrait
http://www.hhs.gov/familyhistory

The U.S. Surgeon General's Family History Initiative encourages all American families to learn more about their health history by filling out a Family Health Portrait online or on paper. Then share the portrait with your healthcare professionals and other family members. Participation is free and your privacy will be protected.

Fit Day Diet and Weight Loss Journal
http://www.fitday.com

This free online diet and weight loss journal helps you keep track of your daily caloric intake, exercise, weight loss, and goals.

Women

Here you'll find sites crammed with health and fitness information especially for women.

MedlinePlus
http://www.nlm.nih.gov/medlineplus/womenshealthissues.html

Browse links to news and articles about women's health issues from the U.S. National Library of Medicine and the National Institutes of Health. Available in Spanish.

The National Women's Health Information Center
http://www.womenshealth.gov/

This site from the Office of Women's Health in the U.S. Department of Health and Human Services offers reliable, current, and free information about women's health issues. Find publications, health news, tools, statistics, organizations, and a calendar of women's health events.

Women's Health Kit
http://www.pueblo.gsa.gov/press/nfcwomenshealthkit06.htm

The FDA's Office of Women's Health and the Federal Citizen Information Center are offering a free kit of ten health publications. Topics include heart disease, over-the-counter drugs, dietary supplements, strokes, lung cancer, cosmetics, even Botox. Print or read online or call (888) 878-3256 to order.

Index

A

accountability, 208, 215
action plans, 209, 214, 224
aging, 26
alcohol, 224
American Council on Exercise, 98
American Medical Association, 59
Arnett, Kerry, 140, 180
assets, 18
Ayala, David, 115–117

B

back pain, 161
Baggett, Julie, 184–185
Baggett, Rod, 184–185
Bailey, Eric, 142, 155
Beavers, Laura, 106–107
Bedwell, Ruth, 126
benefits of fitness, 18, 19
Boothby, Dale, 135
breakfast, 221
Buckmaster, Sandee, 117
buttermilk, 224

C

caffeine, 224
calories, 16
cancer risk, 51
carbohydrates, 168
Carville, Mike, 121–122. *See also*
    Nevada County Meltdown
cheese, 225
chewing gum, 225
childhood obesity, 105–106
choices, 13

cholesterol, 98
"Chose to Move" program, 59
Cicatelli, Greg, 98–99
clothing, 55, 79, 223
commitment, 69–70, 206, 216
community fitness. *See also* Nevada
    County Meltdown
    epidemic of fitness, 212–213
    shifts in behavior, 213–214
    steps toward, 214–216
    where to start, 212
companions, 48, 50
conditioning the mind, 133–134
Conroy, Sean, 111–112
Cooke, Gary, 126
core strength, 161
Countdown with Keith Olbermann,
    158–161, 165
Couric, Katie, 156, 163–165
Currie, Asia, 83
Currie, Chip, 83

D

Daggett, Suzie, 127
Davidson, Peggy, 94–96
deciding on fitness, 206
Dempsey, Bill, 143
denial/honesty, 208
diaries, 16
diets/dieting, 178–179, 202
dining out, 224
discipline, 95, 111–112
Durham Dolls, 182, 185–186

E

Early Show, The, 181, 188
eating, healthful, 168–169
Elliott, Jillian, 157, 164–165
emotional discomfort, 93, 223–224
encouragement, 210
enjoyment, 224
enlightened eating, 13–14
entertaining, 224–225
excuses, 72
exercise
    amount of, 72
    back injury, 161
    caloric expenditure, 150–151
    home gyms, 172
    planning a program, 207
    recovery time, 98–99
    regular, 35, 37
    strength training/cardiovascular,
        133–134

F

failure
    "diets," 17
    fear of, 12
    rates of, 59–60
fast food, 35, 225
fat metabolism, 150
fats (shortening), 168, 222
financial issues, 25–26, 28
fitness. *See also* community fitness
    guidelines, 13
    importance of, 87
    key to, 113
    promoting, 209–210
    steps to, 205–210
fluids, 13
food preparation, 13, 225
Ford, Erma, 44
Frank, Lori Burkart, 126, 128
French eating habits, 33–37
fun, 201–202

G

Glithero, Carolyn, 151
goals, 12, 207–208
Gott, Peter, 178
grains, 225
Grassick, Lorene, 177–178
grocery shopping, 225

H

healthful eating, 168–169
health issues
    injuries, 25–26
    medical supervision, 68
    negative side-effects of dieting,
        178–179
    problems of obesity, 150–151
    reasons for pursuing, 46
    risks of exercise, 85–86
Hillerman, Fred, 100–101
home gyms, 172
honesty/denial, 208
hunger, 222, 223

I

individualism/integration, 202

J

Jackson, Scott, 171–172
Jonsen, Margaret, 113–114, 115
journal-keeping, 208, 223

K

Katis, Jon, 145–146
Kitir, Sirci, 149
Klein, Betty, 117
Koumb, Tim, 117

L

label reading, 224
Lauer, Matt, 164
law of unintended consequences,
    143–144

Lawson, Ranee, 164
learning curve, 209
lifestyle changes, 51–52, 69–70, 72, 150–151, 168–169, 178–179
Lossman, Fred, 146, 159
Lossman, Gayle, 4

M
magical thinking, 179–180
Mallery, Robin Wright, 150
Malthan, Mimi, 81–83
meat, 223
medical supervision, 68
medications, 224
Mediterranean diet, 35
meltdown project. *See* Nevada County Meltdown
"Meltdown Song, The," 185
metabolism, 150–151
Michalski, Susan, 88–89
Moore, Jeannie, 153

N
needs, of others, 105
Nevada County Meltdown. *See also* community fitness
    elements of, 200–203
    evaluations, 199–200
    finale event, 183–186
    ground rules, 134–135
    management structure, 146
    media coverage, 155–156, 158–161, 173–174
    national attention, 161–162
    origins, 121–122
    participants, 132–133, 139, 147, 151–154, 167–168, 176–177
    planning, 123–130
    sharing stories, 149
Nick, Dena, 149
No Diet Zone, 179
nuts, 224

O
Olbermann, Keith, 158–161, 165

P
Palmer, Kathy, 146–147
Personal Wellness Profile, 51
perspective, 111–112
Picture Perfect Weight Loss (Shapiro), 168
planning your actions, 209, 224
portions, 13, 223
professional human beings, 141–142
program schedule, 10
progress reports, 11, 15, 19, 23, 27, 31, 36, 41, 45, 49, 53, 62, 67, 71, 75
project management, 208
promoting fitness, 209–210
protein, 168, 221, 223

R
reasons for eating, 60
reasons for weight loss, 69
recording your food, 223
Redfearn, Dixie, 128
rest, 97–99, 223
restaurants, 225

S
Sakai, Emi, 143–144
salad dressings, 224
Seeman, Laura, 168–169
Seivert, John, 160–161
self-care, 107
self-criticism, 20
self-image, 79, 141
self-indulgence, 93
self-medication, 224
Shapiro, Howard, 168
Sharkey, Cyd, 117
shopping for groceries, 225
Simmons, Jim, 117
skipping meals, 222
sleep deprivation, 98

Smith, Barbara, 164
snacks, 221, 222
sour cream, 224
steps to personal fitness, 205–210
success
  celebrating, 215–216
  overall benefits, 73–76
  reasons for, 63
sugar substitutes, 223
support systems, 124, 206–207, 214

T
Take Five cookbook (Weight Watchers),
  186
telling the truth, 206
temptation, 55–56, 92, 94
thought processes, 114
timing of meals/snacks, 13, 221
Today, 156, 157, 163–165, 181,
  188–189
trans fats, 168
travel issues, 63–68, 92
Turner, Sharyn, 137

U
unintended consequences, law of,
  143–144

V
variety, 223
volume, 221

W
Wagner, Debbie, 51
water, 222
Web site resources, 225–234
weighing routine, 222
weightlifting, 21–22
weight loss plan, 207
well-being, 111
whole grains, 225

Y
yoga, 47
"youthing" versus aging, 81–82

Acknowledgments

Our community is blessed with remarkable physical beauty—lakes, mountains, gently rolling hills, green farmland, towering pine trees, snow-capped mountains, and four gorgeous, constantly changing seasons. Even more impressive, though, are the people here.

Acknowledgment is made to the following individuals and organizations for supporting efforts to make Nevada County "the fittest little county in the nation." Were I to describe what each contributed, I would need to write a second book. Enormously generous, they gave precious time, prizes, expertise, services, and creativity. Without their gifts, the Meltdown would never have occurred, nor this story told.

Many of the individuals who gave support remain anonymous, so my list is incomplete. For those whose names are missing—as well as those I've identified—please accept my heartfelt thanks for your unique, spontaneous gifts and enthusiastic participation. Working together, we created an extraordinary experience for members of our community.

Thank you to Jeff Ackerman; Dayna Amboy; Kerry Arnett; David Ayala; Dr. Paul Auerbach; Dennis Babson; Rod and Julie Baggett; Eric Bailey; Doreen Baldock; Danielle Bandy; Heather Bandy; Shauna Bandy; Judi Bannister; Mary Baron; Laura Beavers; Ruth Bedwell; Drew Bedwell; Nick Bodley; Dale Boothby; Margaret Boothby; Charlie Brock; Carolie Brennan; Pat Butler; Mardie Caldwell; Bill Carlquist; Dick Carson; Mike Carville; Phil Carville; Art Chappell; Greg Cicatelli; Mary Collier; Sean Conroy; Gary Cooke; Beverly Cooper; Carolyn Crane; Chip Currie; Suzie Daggett; Peggy Davidson; Bill Dempsey; Eve Diamond; Richard DicKard; Dr. Linda Foshagen; Robyn Eidson; Jillian Elliott; Ruth Fisher; Molly Fisk; Dave Forsythe; Lori Burkart Frank; Susan Franske; Steve Fraser; Terry Gannon; Sabrina Giner; Jean-Louis Giner; Carolyn Glithero; Arnold

Goldberg; Donna Goldberg; Lorene Grassick; Kady Guyton; John Hart; Sara Heinzel; Dr. Roger Hicks; Fred Hillerman; Cynthia Hubert; Bruce Ivy; Scott Jackson; Barbie Jackson; Sandie "Jake" Jacobson; Barbara Jepsen; Carol Judd; Kathryn Kaiser; Jon Katis; Kitty Kelly, RN, FNP; Ron Kenner; Sirci Kitir; Sue Knopf; Susan Kopp; Dr. Rene Kronland; Sam Kuo; Ranee Lawson; Jim Lea; Sherry Leasure; Kathy Lenk; Martha Lenthe; Muffin Letham; Kris Lienhart; Fred Lossman; Gayle Lossman; Elizabeth Lurie; Marc Lurie; Steve Lurie; Lynn Maas; Paul Mahler; Joni Mahler; Robin Wright Mallery, RN; Mimi Malthan; Julie Marlay; Carol Marquis; Terence McAteer; Scott McIntosh; Wanda McIntosh; Brenda McNeill; Bonnie Metcalf; Wendy Meyers; Susan Michalski; Lynn Miller; Ann Mitchell; Gary Mitchell; Dave Moller; Jeannie Moore; Mary Ann Mueller; Sue Munson; Jennifer Murray; Jan Nagler; Brenda Nascimento; Helen Neff; Dr. Christine Newsom; Dena Nick; Janine Nugent; Jo Nunnink; Janice O'Brien; Kathy Palmer; Jim Perkins; Robin Phillips; Sherry Picciano; Amy Pistone; Dale Pistone; Jamie Porter; R. D. Porter; Alisha Randall; Peggy Raymond; Marianne Reagan; Dixie Redfearn; Judy Richardson; Susan Rice; Helga Rohl; Lore Ross; Linda Rush; Martha Rust, RN; Emi Sakai; Nancy Sanders; Bonnie Schlesinger; Cynthia Schuetz; Ed Scofield; Larry Scott; Laura Seeman, RD; John Seivert, PT; Kathy Sheffield; Jim Simmons; Jennifer Litton Singer; Lew Sitzer; Keely Smith; Pastor Jerry Smith; Pastor Barbara Smith; Toni Souzi; Diedra Spohler; Rita Stevens; Michael Stone; Susan Stone; Amelia Strasler; Patricia Stuckey; Lisa Swarthout; Lindsey Tanner; Amanda Temple; Maxine Tomisser; John Tomisser; Susanna Trevena; Dr. Barry Turner; Sharyn Turner, RN; Dale and Dorothy Volker; Debbie Wagner, RN; Garret Walther; Carole Ward; Patti Wood; Lori Woodhall; Wendi Yellin; Curtis Yew.

The following businesses, organizations, clubs, and government agencies contributed to the Meltdown. Thanks go to Accent Lighting; Alternative Fitness Yoga and Pilates; American Cancer Society; Anytime Fitness; Alternative Fitness Center; Bel Capelli Beauty Salon; Bikram Yoga; Bruce Ivy Construction; Charlie's Angels Café; Cirino's; City of Grass Valley; City of Grass Valley Parks Department; City of Nevada City; Club Sierra Sports and Fitness; Coldwell-Banker Grass Roots Realty; Community Wellness Coalition; Conscious Dream Facilitator;

Courthouse Athletic Club; Courtyard Suites; Curves; Dance Fitness Salon; Durham School Services; Fast and Fit; FCAT; 49er Rotary Club; Friendship Club; Grass Valley and Nevada County Chamber of Commerce; Grass Valley Methodist Church; Helga's Uptown Beauty Salon and Boutique; Highland Llama Trekkers; Interfaith Food Ministry; Jazzercise; KNCO Newstalk; KNCO Star; KVMR Community Radio; Medical Benefits Administration; Mill Street Clothing Co.; Moving Ground; Nevada City Chamber of Commerce; Nevada City Methodist Church; Nevada County Board of Supervisors; Nevada County Fairgrounds; Nevada County Television; Nevada Joint Union High School District Staff; Nevada Irrigation District; Phillips School of Massage; Real Life Fitness; Red Hat Society; Ridge Racquet Club; the *Sacramento Bee*; Seivert Physical Therapy; Sierra Nevada Memorial Hospital; South Yuba Club; SPD Markets; St. Moritz Medical Center Inc.; Synergy Pilates and Massage Center; Tess's Kitchen Store; 3R Elementary School students; TOPS; Trolley Junction Restaurant; the *Union*; United Way; V'Tae Parfum and Body Care; Weight Watchers; Yuba Docs.

We hope our example of individuals and organizations coming together for a common good—to become healthier and more fit—will serve as a model to communities everywhere.

About the Author

Just before turning sixty, Carole Carson decided to re-invent herself. After chronicling her transformation from butterball to butterfly in weekly newspaper articles, Carole invited others to join the fun. Inspired by her example, more than a thousand ordinary people teamed up to lose nearly four tons of fat in two months.

Carole's multifaceted background includes business leadership, marketing, public relations, event planning, writing, training, and consulting to businesses and nonprofits. She drew upon the full range of her experience to make the northern California community fitness event successful. Carole's mission is to communicate her empowering message: "You and your friends can have fun, get fit, and lose weight!"

Carole writes a featured newspaper column, and her articles are available through her Web site at www.HoundPress.com. She has appeared on NBC's *Today* show, CBS's *The Early Show*, MSNBC's *Countdown*, CNN news, and national radio. Besides teaching and consulting, Carole has produced a weekly community television show, *The Tipping Point*, and a reality show, *Go Fat to Fit*.

Programs Available from the Fat to Fit Team

For Individuals

Do you need help finding your own unique way to lose weight and become fit and trim? Are you looking for tools, information, and support as you make the transition? Do you want help identifying local resources that you can use to build your personal fitness program? Will you need ongoing monitoring and coaching?

The **Fat to Fit** team is designed to meet your individual needs. We can provide as much or as little support as you request. Services include consultation and goal setting as well as online monitoring and coaching.

For Organizers

Are you ready to take a public stand for fitness? Are you willing to provide leadership that will make a difference in your community? Do you need support, technical assistance, and tools to achieve maximum impact for your efforts? Will you need encouragement, support, and advice as you go through the exhilarating process? Do you need help tailoring an event for your specific community, whether it's a church, workplace, family, or social group?

The **Fat to Fit** team can provide the specific level of support you need. Services include

- planning
- publicity
- resource acquisition
- programs
- systems
- policies
- speakers
- postevent evaluations

Who Are the Members of the Fat to Fit Team?

The team is a consortium of highly committed individuals who are from diverse professional disciplines and who are united by a passion for promoting fitness. The team may involve a personal trainer, dietitian, wellness counselor, nurse, physical therapist, physician, motivational speaker, or pediatrician, depending upon the nature of your goals.

You or your group may choose to be mentored on an ongoing basis or set up a "consulting as needed" arrangement—a cafeteria-style approach that allows you to choose which services you need and which tasks you can perform independently.
Fees vary based on the kind of services requested.

You may reach us by:

E-MAIL . . . . Fat2Fit@HoundPress.com
PHONE . . . . 🖋 . . . (530) 478-5709
FAX . . . . (530) 478-1108
WEB SITE . . . . .www.HoundPress.com